self-assessment of current knowledge in

Neurology

third edition

811 multiple choice questions
and referenced explanatory answers

Edited By

ARMIN F. HAERER, M.D.
Professor of Neurology
University of Mississippi Medical Center
Jackson, Mississippi

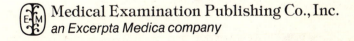 Medical Examination Publishing Co., Inc.
an Excerpta Medica company

notice

The editor(s) and/or author(s) and the publisher of this book have made every effort to ensure that all therapeutic modalities that are recommended are in accordance with accepted standards at the time of publication.

The drugs specified within this book may not have specific approval by the Food and Drug Administration in regard to the indications and dosages that are recommended by the editor(s) and/or author(s). The manufacturer's package insert is the best source of current prescribing information.

Contributors

JOSE BEBIN, M.D., Ph.D., Professor, Department of Pathology; Associate Professor, Department of Neurology, University of Mississippi Medical Center, Jackson, Mississippi

ROBERT D. CURRIER, M.D., Professor and Chairman, Department of Neurology, University of Mississippi Medical Center, Jackson, Mississippi

DURISALA DESAIAH, Ph.D., Assistant Professor, Department of Neurology, University of Mississippi Medical Center, Jackson, Mississippi

MICHAL A. DOUGLAS, M.D., Assistant Professor, Department of Neurology, University of Mississippi Medical Center, Jackson, Mississippi

ARMIN F. HAERER, M.D., Professor, Department of Neurology, University of Mississippi Medical Center, Jackson, Mississippi

GWENDOLYN R. HOGAN, M.D., Professor, Department of Pediatrics; Associate Professor, Department of Neurology, University of Mississippi Medical Center, Jackson, Mississippi

JAN E. JORDAN, M.D., Director, EEG Laboratory, Veterans Administration Hospital; Assistant Professor, Department of Neurology, University of Mississippi Medical Center, Jackson, Mississippi

SHRI K. MISHRA, M.D., Chief, Neurology Service, Veterans Administration Hospital; Associate Professor, Department of Neurology, University of Mississippi Medical Center, Jackson, Mississippi

J. LARRY PARKER, M.D., Assistant Professor, Department of Neurology; Assistant Professor, Division of Ophthalmology, University of Mississippi Medical Center, Jackson, Mississippi

WILLIAM F. RUSSELL, M.D., Assistant Professor, Department of Neurology; Assistant Professor, Department of Radiology, University of Mississippi Medical Center, Jackson, Mississippi

NELL J. RYAN, M.D., Associate Professor, Department of Neurology; Associate Professor, Department of Pediatrics, University of Mississippi Medical Center, Jackson, Mississippi

EDWARD E. SMITH, M.D., Assistant Professor, Department of Pathology; Instructor, Department of Neurology, University of Mississippi Medical Center, Jackson, Mississippi

ANCEL C. TIPTON, Jr., M.D., Assistant Professor, Department of Neurology, University of Mississippi Medical Center, Jackson, Mississippi

Contents ════════════════════════════

Preface

The present edition of **Self-Assessment of Current Knowledge in Neurology** represents a new format that is in keeping with other self-assessment texts of recent years. Brief explanations of the correct choices are provided with the answers in an attempt to enhance the teaching value of the questions. Approximately two-thirds of the questions are referenced, half of these from a variety of recent journals in the general field of Neurology and the other half taken from current texts. The remaining third of the questions are "experience" questions provided by the contributors.

An effort has been made to keep the questions, which are of variable degrees of difficulty, relevant to patient care. Material has been divided into nine chapters representing subareas of Neurology, but some overlap between them is unavoidable. We have made every effort to verify the accuracy of the answers but, because of the number involved, an occasional error may have occurred, for which we apologize in advance. A post-test of 100 multiple choice questions drawn from the material in this text is also included.

We would appreciate comments and suggestions for improving the teaching value of this type of text in the future.

Armin F. Haerer, M.D.
Editor

I: GENERAL NEUROLOGY

PART 1

FOR QUESTIONS 1-14, A STATEMENT IS FOLLOWED BY
FOUR POSSIBLE ANSWERS. ANSWER BY USING THE FOL-
LOWING KEY:

- A. If 1, 2 and 3 are correct
- B. If 1 and 3 are correct
- C. If 2 and 4 are correct
- D. If only 4 is correct
- E. If all 4 are correct

1. Primary intracerebral hemorrhage
    1. has an incidence of about 2 per 100,000 population per year
    2. is more common in females than in males
    3. decreases after age 50
    4. has decreased gradually in incidence during the past 30 years
    REF: Ann. Neurol. 5:367, 1979

2. Computed tomography of the brain in patients with CNS lupus demonstrates
    1. sulcal enlargement is most common
    2. subdural hematomas are nearly as common as infarcts
    3. ventricular enlargement is common
    4. infarcts and intracerebral hemorrhages are rare
    REF: Ibid., p. 158

3. Regarding human brain weights
    1. male and female brain weights are nearly equal
    2. the largest increase in brain weight occurs during the first 3 years of life
    3. brain weight begins to decline at 25 years of age
    4. brain weights are some 10% lower during the ninth dec-ade than during the early adult life
    REF: Ann. Neurol. 4:345, 1978

1

4.   Effects of phenytoin on bone and vitamin D metabolism
       include
       1.   decrease in serum calcium
       2.   decrease in serum albumin
       3.   decrease in serum 25-hydroxycholecalciferol
       4.   increase in serum alkaline phosphatase
       REF: Ann. Neurol. 5:374, 1979

5.   Facial myokymia
       1.   is an intermittent twitching of muscles of the face
       2.   is less common than myokymia of the upper extremity
       3.   is most often seen with polyradiculoneuropathy
       4.   is associated with multiple sclerosis or brain stem
            neoplasms
       REF: Neurology 29:662, 1979

6.   Unilateral neglect (hemi-inattention) may result from le-
       sions in the
       1.   parietal lobe
       2.   putamen
       3.   cingulate gyrus
       4.   thalamus
       REF: Ibid. , p. 690

7.   Calcification of the basal ganglia found on computerized
       tomography
       1.   is usually asymmetric
       2.   involves mainly the putamen
       3.   rarely involves the globus pallidus
       4.   has little pathophysiologic significance of altered cal-
            cium metabolism
       REF: Ibid. , p. 328

8.   Regarding risk factors for cerebral complications of
       angiography for transient ischemic attacks and stroke
       1.   patients in whom the study is most needed tend to be
            those at greatest risk from it
       2.   risk is unrelated to the number of selective injections
       3.   risk is strongly related to the number of previous tran-
            sient ischemic attacks
       4.   the degree of arterial stenosis does not affect the risk
       REF: Ibid. , p. 4

9. In response to a standardized prolonged exercise test
    1. the correlation of changes in blood lactate, creatine kinase and fatty acids may be of diagnostic usefulness
    2. patients with a disproportionate rise in creatine kinase may have metabolic myopathies
    3. patients with a disproportionate rise of lactate may have mitochondrial abnormalities
    4. normals do not show a rise of lactate or creatine kinase
    REF: Ibid. , p. 636

10. Wernicke's encephalopathy is
    1. usually diagnosed antemortem
    2. associated with thiamin deficiency
    3. not associated with abnormal liver function tests
    4. usually not diagnosed during life
    REF: J. Neurol. , Neurosurg. and Psych. 42:226, 1979

11. Partial seizures with complex symptomatology
    1. are also known as psychomotor seizures
    2. respond best to ethosuximide
    3. respond about equally to carbamazepine as to phenytoin
    4. should never be treated with temporal lobectomy
    REF: Tyler, H. R. , Dawson, D. M. , eds. : Current Neurology, vol. 1, Houghton Mifflin, Boston, 1978, p. 247

12. Regarding anticonvulsants
    1. trimethadione is effective for grand mal attacks
    2. valproate is effective for petit mal and some grand mal attacks
    3. phenytoin is rapidly effective if given intramuscularly
    4. primidone is partially metabolized to phenobarbital
    REF: Ibid. , pp. 247-252

13. Vincristine
    1. almost always causes a peripheral neuropathy
    2. spares the autonomic nervous system as a rule
    3. therapy may be accompanied by seizures but the causal relationship is unclear
    4. has an effective antidote to minimize toxicity from it
    REF: Ibid. , pp. 307-311

14. A 70-year-old woman with a blood pressure of 160/105 entered the hospital 12 hours after a left hemiparesis, which had lasted 2 hours. As you examine her the hemiparesis begins again. Would you
    1. request an immediate arteriogram
    2. request an immediate CT scan
    3. do an LP and if it showed no blood, proceed to give heparin
    4. start aspirin therapy and reduce her blood pressure medically

FOR EACH OF THE FOLLOWING MULTIPLE CHOICE QUES-
TIONS, SELECT THE ONE MOST APPROPRIATE ANSWER:

15. Generalized wasting in patients with carcinomas is usually
    A. neurogenic
    B. myogenic
    C. the Eaton-Lambert syndrome
    D. secondary to a myelitis
    E. none of these
    REF: Brain 101:53, 1978

16. Involvement of the trigeminal sensory root may be a false localizing sign because of
    A. a displaced brainstem
    B. the angulation of the root as it enters the posterior fossa
    C. extrinsic tumors (usually)
    D. all of these
    E. none of these
    REF: Ibid., p. 119

17. Neurologic signs are present in intermittent claudication of the cauda equina
    A. only at rest
    B. only with exercise
    C. at rest and worsened with exercise
    D. only during the first weeks of the disease
    E. only late in the disease
    REF: Ibid., p. 211

18. Surgical therapy for intermittent claudication of the cauda equina is
    A. an emergency
    B. often successful and to be recommended
    C. contraindicated
    D. still experimental
    E. impossible at this time
    REF: Ibid., p. 211

19. Somatosensory seizures are
    A. usually simple seizures
    B. usually complex seizures
    C. rarely associated with Jacksonian fits
    D. without localizing value
    E. ipsilateral to the lesion
    REF: Ibid. , p. 307

20. Muscle weakness and wasting in the thoracic outlet syndrome is most common in the
    A. biceps
    B. forearm
    C. hand
    D. shoulder
    E. A and D
    REF: Brain 100:601, 1977

21. Cerebral ischemic events within the territory of an occluded artery
    A. appear to be mainly local thrombotic episodes
    B. appear to be mainly of embolic origin
    C. may arise from the "stump" of the internal carotid artery
    D. A and C
    E. B and C
    REF: Stroke 9:448, 1978

22. Which statement is not true regarding cerebral infarction in young adults?
    A. Two-thirds of patients will recover or improve to functional independence
    B. Premature atherosclerotic disease and hypertension play a role
    C. Cerebral embolism of cardiac origin is a frequent cause
    D. The etiology can be identified in over half of the cases
    E. Occlusive extracranial vascular disease is the leading cause
    REF: Ibid. , p. 39

23. The use of corticosteroids to combat cerebral edema in stroke
    A. is possibly useful in large infarctions
    B. provides an increase in survival in most controlled studies
    C. is fairly well understood in terms of their cellular effect to reduce edema
    D. all of these
    E. none of these
    REF: Stroke 10:68, 1979

24. The results of carotid endarterectomy vary with
    A. the surgeon
    B. the institution
    C. the preoperative status of the patient
    D. all of these
    E. none of these
    REF: Ibid. , p. 117

25. As treatment in the acute phase of stroke, which of the following were useful?
    A. Hydergine R
    B. A corticosteroid
    C. Mannitol
    D. All of these
    E. None of these
    REF: Stroke 9:130, 1978

26. Risk factors for stroke include
    A. transient ischemic attacks
    B. polycythemia
    C. amaurosis fugax
    D. hypertension
    E. all of these
    REF: Ibid. , p. 299

27. Benign rolandic paroxysmal epilepsy of children
    A. is 5-7 times as frequent as petit mal epilepsy and accounts for 25% of all childhood epilepsy
    B. Has stereotyped spike foci in central and midtemporal areas on EEG
    C. has a favorable prognosis for complete cure (whether treated or untreated) by age 13
    D. has frequent neuropsychiatric abnormalities associated with it
    E. A, B and C
    REF: Epilepsia 19:337, 1978

28. Magnesium sulfate anticonvulsant effect is similar to that produced by
    A. phenobarbital
    B. phenytoin
    C. primidone
    D. all of these
    E. none of these
    REF: Ibid. , p. 88

29. Palatal myoclonus following brainstem infarction begins at a median interval of
    A. 5 days after infarction
    B. 2 weeks after infarction
    C. 6 weeks after infarction
    D. 10 months after infarction
    E. none of these
    REF: Ann. Neurol. 5:72, 1979

30. The most common side effect of valproic acid is
    A. gastrointestinal upset
    B. loss of hair
    C. aplastic anemia
    D. excessive sedation
    E. none of these
    REF: Ann Neurol. 3:20, 1978

31. Speech disorders develop most commonly with lesions of the cerebellar
    A. right hemisphere
    B. left hemisphere
    C. vermis
    D. inferior surface
    E. superior surface
    REF: Ibid., p. 285

32. The prognosis in transverse myelopathy is best with
    A. an acute onset
    B. severe early back pain
    C. a subacute onset
    D. preceding febrile illness
    E. B and D
    REF: Ann Neurol. 4:51, 1978

33. The most common neurologic involvement in Paget disease is in
    A. cranial nerve VII
    B. cranial nerve VIII
    C. spinal cord
    D. spinal roots and nerves
    E. none of these
    REF: Neurology 29:448, 1979

34. The risk of developing epilepsy by age 20 for a child who has experienced a febrile convulsion is
    A. 6%
    B. 20%
    C. 2.5%
    D. 1%
    E. 30%
    REF: Ibid., p. 297

35. The most common location of headache in children with migraine is
    A. bilateral frontal
    B. unilateral frontal
    C. posterior
    D. bilateral temporal
    E. unilateral temporal
    REF: Ibid., p. 507

36. Which may be useful in the treatment of hereditary paroxysmal ataxia?
    A. Carbamazepine
    B. Acetazolamide
    C. Propranolol
    D. All of these
    E. None of these
    REF: Neurology 28:1259, 1978

37. Intravenous phenytoin in a dose of 18 mg per kilogram maintains serum levels above 10 micrograms per milliliter for
    A. 12 hours
    B. 24 hours
    C. 48 hours
    D. 72 hours
    E. 120 hours
    REF: Ibid., p. 874

38. Diabetic peripheral nerves are
    A. slightly more sensitive to ischemia than normals
    B. much more sensitive to ischemia
    C. less sensitive to ischemia
    D. the same as non-diabetics in sensitivity to ischemia
    E. none of these
    REF: Neurology 29:695, 1979

39. 4-aminopyridine gives improvement in muscular strength and neuromuscular transmission in
    A. human myasthenia gravis
    B. experimental botulism
    C. the Eaton-Lambert syndrome
    D. all of these
    E. none of these
    REF: J. Neurol., Neurosurg., Psychiat. 42:171, 1979

40. Angiomas of the spinal cord
    A. usually are on the dorsum of the cord
    B. occur most often in middle-aged women
    C. are symptomatically but not functionally improved by operation
    D. all of these
    E. A and C only
    REF: Ibid., p. 1

41. The Tolosa-Hunt syndrome
    A. is usually the result of nonspecific granulomatous infiltration of the carotid artery
    B. does not usually relapse and remit
    C. usually responds rapidly to steroids
    D. should be surgically explored
    E. all of these
    REF: Ibid., p. 270

42. The consistent features of capsular infarcts include
    A. a purely motor hemiparesis
    B. hemiparesis plus sensory loss
    C. hemiparesis plus homonymous hemianopsia
    D. hemiparesis with prolonged aphasia (in dominant hemisphere)
    E. C and D only
    REF: Arch. Neurol. 36:73, 1979

43. Focal motor and generalized epilepsy treatment with carbamazepine or phenytoin showed
    A. better seizure control with carbamazepine
    B. more acute side effects with carbamazepine
    C. better seizure control with phenytoin
    D. more acute side effects with phenytoin
    E. none of these
    REF: Ibid., p. 22

44. The lesion in ataxic hemiparesis is in the
    A. ipsilateral cerebellar hemisphere
    B. contralateral cerebellar hemisphere
    C. medulla
    D. ipsilateral basis pontis
    E. contralateral basis pontis
    REF: Arch. Neurol.35:126, 1978

45. Regional cerebral blood flow in the hemispheres with psychophysiologic activation
    A. increases in normal persons
    B. remains the same over ischemic hemispheres in stroke patients
    C. decreases in epileptics
    D. remains unchanged in demented persons
    E. A, B and D
    REF: Ibid. , p. 350

46. Bilingual persons
    A. have both languages represented in the center of the language area of the dominant cortex
    B. have each language represented in totally separate areas of the cortex
    C. have certain sites involved in only one of the languages
    D. A and C
    E. none of these
    REF: Ibid. , p. 409

47. Antibody response to arboviruses is increased in
    A. multiple sclerosis
    B. amyotrophic lateral sclerosis
    C. equine encephalitis
    D. all of these
    E. none of these
    REF: Ibid. , p. 440

48. The principal long-term residuals of Jamaica ginger paralysis are
    A. spasticity and other upper motor neuron signs
    B. hyporeflexia and lower motor neuron signs
    C. marked sensory deficit
    D. severe dementia
    E. none of these
    REF: Ibid. , p. 530

49. Which is the least likely feature of early Huntington's disease?
    A. Low IQ
    B. Impaired memory quotients
    C. Impaired short-term memory
    D. Impaired retrieval from long-term memory
    E. Choreiform movements
    REF: Ibid., p. 585

50. Regional cerebral blood flow in aphasia patients shows abnormalities in
    A. Broca's area consistently, with motor (nonfluent) aphasia
    B. superior-posterior temporal cortex consistently, with sensory (fluent) aphasia
    C. lower rolandic and superior-posterior temporal cortex consistently, with global aphasia
    D. A and B
    E. B and C
    REF: Ibid., p. 625

51. For patients with intracranial metastatic neoplasms
    A. no single treatment modality was clearly better than another
    B. any form of therapy was superior to no treatment at all
    C. the prognosis with a solitary metastasis from known primaries was much better than for multiple metastases
    D. A and B only
    E. B and C only
    REF: Ibid., p. 754

52. Choline and lecithin have been said to be helpful in the treatment of
    A. Huntington's disease
    B. Friedreich's ataxia
    C. presenile dementia
    D. all of these
    E. none of these
    REF: N. Engl. J. Med. 300:1113, 1979 (letter to the editor)

53. Interferon in the treatment of herpes zoster has been shown to
    A. be of no effect
    B. provide complete cure
    C. limit visceral complications
    D. B and C
    E. none of these
    REF: N. Engl. J. Med. 298:981, 1978

54. In hypsarrhythmia (salaam attacks) ACTH may improve
    A. the EEG abnormalities
    B. seizure control
    C. associated mental retardation
    D. all of these
    E. none of these
    REF: Clin. EEG 7:149, 1976

55. A lesion of the middle trunk of the brachial plexus is essentially a
    A. C-6 root lesion
    B. C-7 root lesion
    C. C-5, C-6 root lesion
    D. C-8, T-1 root lesion
    E. none of these
    REF: Mayo Clinic Proc. 53:801, 1978

56. In measles encephalitis clinical and EEG improvement results from
    A. norepinephrine
    B. prostaglandins
    C. enkephalins
    D. L-dopa
    E. eserine
    REF: Eur. Neurol. 17:265, 1978

57. In the determination of cerebral death, the echoencephalogram can supplement the EEG by showing
    A. a loss of all echos
    B. evidence of lateral ventricle enlargement
    C. spurious location of echos
    D. a loss of midline pulsations
    E. random noise
    REF: J. Neurosurg. 48:866, 1978

58. Which statement is true for acute intermittent porphyric neuropathy?
    A. This is an axonal neuropathy
    B. It is a demyelinating form of neuropathy
    C. It is primarily a radiculopathy
    D. All of these
    E. None of these
    REF: Muscle and Nerve 1:292, 1978

59. Sleep apnea is associated with
    A. renal disease
    B. cardiac disease
    C. hepatic failure
    D. encephalitis
    E. peripheral neuropathy
    REF: Tex. Med. 73:49, 1977

60. Recovery from the comatose condition is correlated with
    A. the lack of cerebral blood flow
    B. the number of clinical seizures
    C. the length of silent periods between bursts of EEG sup-
       pression bursts
    D. the presence of more than 8 peaks in the somatosen-
       sory evoked potential
    E. none of these
    REF: Exp. Neurol. 60:304, 1978

61. The schizophrenia-like psychosis of epilepsy differs from
    ordinary schizophrenia in that
    A. epilepsy is present
    B. there is usually no psychosis in the immediate family
    C. the EEG shows anterior temporal abnormality
    D. all of these
    E. A and C only
    REF: Pincus, J. H. and Tucker, G. J.: Behavioral Neu-
    rology, 2nd edition, Oxford University Press, New York,
    1978, p. 43

62. The epileptic psychosis has been postulated as being caused
    by
    A. the psychologic reaction to the seizures
    B. the anticonvulsant medications
    C. repeated seizures
    D. "subictal" seizures
    E. all of these
    REF: Ibid., pp. 40-41

63. Hemispheric asymmetries
    A. occur in 65-75% of human brains
    B. support the argument for differential processing ca-
       pacities in the hemispheres
    C. support the argument for attentional differences be-
       tween the hemispheres
    D. A and B
    E. A and C
    REF: Tyler, H. R., Dawson, D. M., eds.: Current Neu-
    rology, vol. 1, Houghton Mifflin, Boston, 1978, p. 341

64. Severe dementia occurs in approximately what percent of the population over age 65?
    A.   1%
    B.   4-5%
    C.   11-12%
    D.   17%
    E.   31%
    REF: Ibid. , p. 361

65. Fatalities from severe cases of senile dementia in the United States average annually near
    A.   2, 000
    B.   20, 000
    C.   100, 000
    D.   200, 000
    E.   2, 000, 000
    REF: Ibid. , p. 362

66. The prevalence of Parkinson's disease in the United States is near
    A.   0. 5 per 1, 000
    B.   2 per 1, 000
    C.   3. 5 per 1, 000
    D.   5 per 1, 000
    E.   none of these
    REF: Ibid. , p. 363

67. The most common clinical findings in patients with Alzheimer's disease, in decreasing order of frequency, are
    A.   memory loss, disorientation, agitation
    B.   agitation, dysphasia, disorientation
    C.   memory loss, dyspraxia, gait disturbance
    D.   agitation, memory loss, dyspraxia
    E.   incontinence, disorientation, memory loss
    REF: Ibid. , p. 365

68. Neurologic complications of cardiac catheterization commonly are of which type and occur in which location?
    A.   Thrombotic, in the right hemisphere
    B.   Hemorrhagic, in the basal ganglia
    C.   Embolic, in the brain stem
    D.   Thrombotic, in the brain stem
    E.   Hemorrhagic, in the left hemisphere
    REF: Ibid. , p. 469

69. With mitral valve prolapse
   A. small strokes occur in nearly one-third of patients
   B. strokes, when they occur, are usually embolic
   C. auricular fibrillation increases the risk of embolism
   D. B and C only
   E. A, B and C
   REF: Ibid., p. 469

70. Which statement is false for patients with migraine?
   A. There is platelet hyperaggregability during the prodrome
   B. Serotonin levels increase with the prodrome
   C. Serotonin levels decrease with the headache
   D. Platelet adhesiveness increases with the headache
   E. Platelet aggregation response to epinephrine increases with the headache
   REF: Ibid., p. 469

71. Features of adrenoleukodystrophy include
   A. pronounced skin pallor
   B. reduced adrenal reserve
   C. probable abnormal fatty acid synthesis
   D. A and B
   E. A, B and C
   REF: Ibid., p. 471

72. Strionigral degeneration
   A. does not respond as well to levodopa as does paralysis agitans
   B. usually presents with an asymmetrical parkinsonian syndrome
   C. may mimic Shy-Drager syndrome
   D. A and C only
   E. A, B and C
   REF: Ibid., p. 113

73. Shy-Drager syndrome and parkinsonism have certain features in common. Which of the following is not true?
   A. Both may have bradykinesia
   B. Both show hypersensitivity to intravenous noradrenaline
   C. Both show hypersensitivity to intravenous dopamine
   D. Fluorocortisone may improve Shy-Drager patients more than parkinsonism
   E. Levodopa is more effective for parkinsonism than for Shy-Drager syndrome
   REF: Ibid., p. 114

74. Hypertensive headache
    A. may occur with acute as well as chronic hypertension
    B. represents a very small percentage of headaches in the general population
    C. has a well understood pathogenesis
    D. A and B
    E. A and C
    REF: Ibid., pp. 197-198

75. Which statement is not true of hypertensive encephalopathy?
    A. It appears to be decreasing in incidence
    B. It is affecting a smaller number of older patients in recent years
    C. Hypertension of whatever cause may produce it
    D. Papilledema is generally proportional to the increase in intracranial pressure
    E. Convulsions are common with this condition
    REF: Ibid., p. 199

76. Which statement is false concerning intracranial aneurysms?
    A. There is a gradual increase in the overall prevalence
    B. They are slightly more common in females
    C. The highest likelihood of rupture is in the sixth decade
    D. About 2% occur in children or adolescents
    E. Surgical treatment has been found superior to conservative management in alert patients, whether adults or children
    REF: Ibid., pp. 223, 236

77. The neurologic complications of 5-fluorouracil therapy
    A. occur in 15-20% of patients with conventional doses of 15 mg/kg
    B. affect mainly the basal ganglia and peripheral nerves
    C. are related to the total dose rather than the dose given at each administration
    D. all of these
    E. none of these
    REF: Ibid., p. 313

78. Spinal epidural abscess
    A. is often associated with a trivial back injury
    B. is rarely associated with fever
    C. is never associated with nuchal rigidity
    D. is associated with a low CSF glucose
    E. all of these
    REF: Adams, R. D. and Victor, M.: Principles of Neurology, McGraw-Hill, New York, 1977, p. 473

79. Cervical spondylosis is often associated with
   A. a painful, stiff neck
   B. shoulder and arm pain
   C. hand atrophy
   D. A, B and C
   E. B and C only
   REF: Ibid., p. 482

80. Syringomyelia
   A. is often associated with craniocervical malformations
   B. is steadily progressive
   C. is very rarely associated with pain
   D. A, B and C
   E. A and C only
   REF: Ibid., p. 487

81. Peripheral neuropathy is primarily interstitial in
   A. leprosy
   B. polyradiculoneuropathy
   C. vaccinogenic neuropathy
   D. all of these
   E. none of these
   REF: Dyck, P. J., Thomas, P. K., Lambert, E. H.:
   Peripheral Neuropathy, vol. I, W. B. Saunders Co., Philadelphia, 1975, p. 332

82. In regard to Dejerine-Sottas disease
   A. it is inherited as an autosomal recessive trait
   B. there is clinical enlargement of various nerves (hypertrophic neuropathy)
   C. there is onionbulb formation
   D. all of these
   E. none of these
   REF: Ibid., p. 856

83. Which of the following may be associated with chronic progressive external ophthalmoplegia (CPEO)?
   A. Retinal degeneration
   B. Cardiac conduction abnormalities
   C. Peripheral neuropathy
   D. A and C only
   E. A, B and C
   REF: Glaser, J. S., Smith, J. L., eds.: Neuro-Ophthalmology, vol. VIII, Symposium of B. P. E. I., C. V. Mosby Co., St. Louis, 1975, pp. 216-236

84. Cerebrospinal fluid in pituitary apoplexy may be
    A. hemorrhagic
    B. pleocytic
    C. normal
    D. all of these
    E. none of these
    REF: Glaser, J. S. , Smith, J. L. , eds. : Neuro-Ophthal-
    mology, Symposium of the University of Miami, C. V.
    Mosby Co. , St. Louis, 1975, pp. 156-157

85. The anterior interosseous nerve syndrome due to entrap-
    ment of this major branch of the median nerve produces
    A. pain in the proximal forearm
    B. paresis or paralysis of the flexor pollicis longus
    C. paresis or paralysis of the flexor profundus 2 and 3
    D. paresis or paralysis of the pronator quadratus
    E. all of these

86. The Aicardi syndrome
    A. is recessive
    B. is dominant
    C. is not hereditary
    D. is due to poisoning with Uranium 235
    E. none of these

87. A 22-year-old white female presented with a one year his-
    tory of withdrawal, peculiar gait and weight loss. Her
    mother had the same difficulty and died in a State Hospital.
    The likely diagnosis is
    A. Wilson's disease
    B. hereditary ataxia
    C. familial parkinsonism
    D. Huntington's disease
    E. none of these

88. A 35-year-old female with chronic migraine is having daily
    severe headaches and is taking an analgesic containing a
    barbiturate, an ergotamine preparation and propranolol,
    each several times a day. As your first step in treatment,
    what would you do?
    A. Increase the ergot preparation
    B. Stop the propranolol and barbiturate-analgesic
       preparation
    C. Increase the propranolol
    D. Stop the ergot and the analgesic mixture
    E. Increase the propranolol and ergot

89. A physician refers to you his mother, who overnight has started to shake in one hand while at rest. He is unfamiliar with parkinsonism starting in this way. This presentation of parkinsonism is
    A. common
    B. less common than onset in a leg
    C. uncommon but not worrisome
    D. so uncommon that the patient should be studied for a focal lesion
    E. none of these

90. Malignant hyperpyrexia may improve with
    A. caffeine
    B. calcium gluconate
    C. dantrolene sodium
    D. all of these
    E. none of these

91. Tardive dyskinesia
    A. may be due to denervation hypersensitivity of dopamine receptors
    B. may improve with resumption of phenothiazines or butyrophenones
    C. consistently improves with deanol
    D. B and C only
    E. A and B only

92. Multiple sclerosis
    A. is usually acquired just before it becomes symptomatic
    B. is caused by a virus recoverable from plaques
    C. is more common in Minnesota than in Louisiana
    D. all of these
    E. none of these

93. In patients with benign intracranial hypertension (pseudo-tumor cerebri)
    A. the ventricular system is usually enlarged
    B. there is usually a good response to corticosteroids
    C. antihypertensive drugs are effective
    D. the funduscopic examination is usually normal
    E. all of these

94. Which is the least effective treatment for tic douloureux?
    A. Phenytoin
    B. Hydergine ^{R}
    C. Carbamazepine
    D. Nerve avulsion
    E. Intracranial nerve section

95. Least likely to occur in patients with Friedreich's ataxia is
    A. diabetes mellitus
    B. kyphoscoliosis
    C. hypothyroidism
    D. cerebellar dysarthria
    E. neurogenic feet

96. Treatable causes of dementia include
    A. pernicious anemia
    B. syphilis
    C. subdural hematoma
    D. hypothyroidism
    E. all of these

97. Catamenial sciatica is caused by
    A. spinal arachnoiditis
    B. subarachnoid hemorrhage
    C. endometriosis
    D. herniated nucleus pulposus
    E. sciatic nerve injections

98. Bell's palsy in pregnancy is
    A. less common than in nonpregnant females
    B. most common in the third trimester and first two postpartum weeks
    C. least common in the third trimester and first two postpartum weeks
    D. most common in the first trimester
    E. most common in the second trimester

99. Postpartum foot drop is caused by
    A. hypotension during delivery
    B. caesarian section with retractor pressure
    C. compression of the lumbosacral trunk by the infant's brow
    D. a painful episiotomy
    E. fatigue

100. The most common presenting symptoms and signs of carcinomatous meningitis are
    A. headache and cranial nerve palsies
    B. cerebellar ataxia and field defects
    C. papilledema and blurred vision
    D. dementias and incontinence
    E. none of these

101. The CSF findings in meningeal carcinomatosis usually
     reveal
     A. normal protein, increased lymphocytes, normal
        glucose
     B. normal protein, normal number of lymphocytes, nor-
        mal glucose
     C. elevated protein, normal number of lymphocytes, nor-
        mal glucose
     D. elevated protein, increased number of lymphocytes,
        decreased glucose
     E. none of these

102. Increased intracranial pressure without specific local-
     izing signs most commonly is due to mass lesions in
     A. the parietal or occipital lobes
     B. the frontal lobe or cerebellum
     C. the sella or ventricles
     D. the brainstem
     E. none of these

103. The syndrome of pseudotumor cerebri most commonly
     occurs in
     A. obese females with menstrual difficulty
     B. obese males with impotence
     C. young females with skin moles
     D. older males with hyperphagia
     E. none of these

104. Glomus tumors often present as a
     A. jugular foramen syndrome
     B. middle ear mass
     C. conductive hearing loss with rhinorrhea
     D. all of these
     E. none of these

105. In chorea gravidarum
     A. the chorea persists indefinitely
     B. it never recurs with subsequent pregnancies
     C. about 35% have a definite history of rheumatic fever
     D. all of these
     E. none of these

106.   The most common nontraumatic cause of subarachnoid
       hemorrhage in women under age 25 is
       A.   ruptured aneurysms
       B.   unknown
       C.   bleeding disorders
       D.   arteriovenous malformations
       E.   none of these

107.   Wilson's disease is treatable with
       A.   tetracycline
       B.   steroids
       C.   propranolol
       D.   penicillamine
       E.   all of these

108.   The effect of amantadine HCl (Symmetrel [R]) in the treat-
       ment of parkinsonism lasts usually
       A.   1- 3 months
       B.   3-12 months
       C.   indefinitely
       REF: Merritt, H. H. : A Textbook of Neurology, 6th ed. ,
       Lea & Febiger, Philadelphia, 1979, p. 525

109.   Volkmann's ischemic process of the forearm frequently
       causes entrapment of the
       A.   median nerve
       B.   radial nerve
       C.   ulnar nerve
       D.   posterior interosseous nerve at the arcade of Frohse
       E.   A and C
       F.   B and D

110.   The prognosis of aphasia
       A.   is best, if untreated, for Broca's and moderate fluent
            types
       B.   is worst, if untreated, for long-standing global and
            Wernicke's types
       C.   is improved similarly in all types with rehabilitation
       D.   is improved the most with rehabilitation for Broca's
            type
       E.   B and D only
       F.   A, B and C only
       REF: Arch. Neurol. 36:190, 1979

111. An important factor in the causation of central pontine myelinolysis is
    A. failure to give supplemental thiamine
    B. contaminants and toxic substances in the alcohol
    C. hyponatremia
    D. cerebral hemisphere edema
    REF: Neurology 29:147, 1979

112. Ophthalmoplegic migraine usually has its onset in
    A. childhood
    B. midadult life
    C. the elderly
    D. none of these
    REF: Ophthalmic Seminars 1:413, 1976

113. The most useful odors for testing olfactory nerve function are
    A. cloves and peppermint
    B. camphor and ammonia
    C. floral and musks
    D. none of these
    REF: Brain 100:377, 1977

114. Friedreich's ataxia is inherited as
    A. autosomal recessive
    B. autosomal dominant
    C. sex linked recessive
    D. none of these
    REF: Dyck, P. J., Thomas, P. K., Lambert, E. H.: Peripheral Neuropathy, vol. II, W. B. Saunders Co., Philadelphia, 1975, p. 816

115. Which of the following diagnostic procedures is most likely to be abnormal in multiple sclerosis?
    A. Eye movement recordings
    B. Computerized tomography scan
    C. Sensory evoked potentials
    D. The EEG

116. Carcinomatous meningitis is most commonly seen with which of the following?
    A. Oat cell carcinoma
    B. Sarcomas
    C. Adenocarcinomas
    D. None of these

117.   The Framingham study shows the greatest risk of stroke
        is with
        A. atrial fibrillation
        B. rheumatic heart disease
        C. atrial fibrillation with rheumatic heart disease
        RE F: Neurology 28:973, 1978

PART 2

FOR QUESTIONS 118-146, A STATEMENT IS FOLLOWED BY FOUR POSSIBLE ANSWERS. ANSWER BY USING THE FOLLOWING KEY:

    A. If only A is correct
    B. If only B is correct
    C. If both A and B are correct
    D. If neither A nor B are correct

118. Regarding cerebral "dominance"
    A. the right or "minor" hemisphere seems dominant for propositional speech
    B. the left hemisphere seems dominant for affective speech
    C. both
    D. neither
    REF: <u>Arch. Neurol</u>. 36:144, 1979

119. Psychosis and seizure disorders occur in
    A. adult onset Gaucher's disease
    B. juvenile onset Gaucher's disease
    C. both
    D. neither
    REF: Ibid. , p. 95

120. Bromocriptine in parkinsonism
    A. improves patients with severe "on-off" disabilities from L-dopa
    B. produces benefits similar to ten times the amount of L-dopa with carbidopa
    C. both
    D. neither
    REF: Ibid. , 35:503

121. The prognosis of amyotrophic lateral sclerosis
    A. is substantially better in those whose disease begins below age 50 than in older onset cases
    B. carries an overall 5-year survival of near 40%
    C. both
    D. neither
    REF: Arch. Neurol. 35:638, 1978

122. Primary pineal tumors
    A. most commonly occur in adolescent boys
    B. usually produce hypothalamic symptoms
    C. both
    D. neither
    REF: Ibid. , p. 736

123. Parkinsonism
    A. improves with naltrexane, an opiate antagonist
    B. improves, including the "on-off" effect, with N-n-propyl-norapomorphine
    C. both
    D. neither
    REF: Ibid. , pp. 787, 810

124. Visual hallucinations as a "release" phenomenon after occipital lobe damage are
    A. immediate in onset
    B. repetitive, and of brief duration
    C. both
    D. neither
    REF: Ann. Neurol. 2:432, 1977

125. Mortality in presenile and senile dementia patients without focal lesions or systemic disease may be predicted by
    A. computerized tomography
    B. EEG and expressive language defects
    C. both
    D. neither
    REF: Ann. Neurol. 3:248, 1978

126. Dialysis dementia or encephalopathy is characterized by
    A. nonfluent speech
    B. abnormal EEG
    C. both
    D. neither
    REF: Ibid. , 4:199

127.   Prosopagnosia (inability to recognize faces) occurs with
         lesions in the
         A.   nondominant occipitotemporal lobes
         B.   bilateral inferior occipitotemporal lobes
         C.   both
         D.   neither
         REF: J. Neurol. , Neurosurg. , Psychiat. 40:395, 1977

128.   The neurologic signs and symptoms of Paget disease are
         due to
         A.   vascular distention
         B.   mechanical impingement
         C.   both
         D.   neither
         REF: Neurology 29:448, 1979

129.   Horizontal gaze nystagmus correlates reliably with
         A.   total phenytoin blood levels
         B.   free phenytoin blood levels
         C.   both
         D.   neither
         REF: Epilepsia 19:96, 1978

130.   Strokes in young adults are often caused by
         A.   unknown factors
         B.   alcoholic excess in a usual nondrinker
         C.   both
         D.   neither
         REF: Stroke 9:39, 1978

131.   Which of the following compounds have been found useful
         in the treatment of acute intermittent porphyria?
         A.   Phenothiazines
         B.   Glucose
         C.   Both
         D.   Neither
         REF: Dyck, P. J. , Thomas, P. K. , Lambert, E. H. :
         Peripheral Neuropathy, vol. II, W. B. Saunders Co. ,
         Philadelphia, 1975, p. 953

132. In normal individuals, study of visual hemi-field presentation demonstrates
    A. English word recognition is better in the right visual field than in the left
    B. face recognition is better in the left visual field than in the right
    C. both
    D. neither
    REF: Tyler, H. R., Dawson, D. M., eds.: Current Neurology, vol. 1, Houghton Mifflin, Boston, 1978, p. 342

133. Creutzfeldt-Jakob disease
    A. has elevated CSF immunoglobulins G and M
    B. usually lasts 3-6 months to death
    C. both
    D. neither

134. Counterimmunoelectrophoresis is helpful in the diagnosis of purulent meningitis because it
    A. identifies the drugs to which the organism is sensitive
    B. rapidly identifies many etiologic agents accurately
    C. both
    D. neither

135. St. Louis encephalitis
    A. is spread by mosquitoes, the reservoir being in birds
    B. responds to vidarabine
    C. both
    D. neither

136. Mirror movements of the hands may be
    A. hereditary and idiopathic
    B. associated with Klippel-Feil deformity
    C. both
    D. neither

137. Regarding cryptococcal meningitis
    A. a quick and reliable method of diagnosis is with the CSF cryptococcal antigen test
    B. flucytosine is the treatment of choice
    C. both
    D. neither

138. A patient suspected of having seizures has a normal EEG. What can you conclude from this?
     A. The patient is faking his seizures
     B. The EEG is of no value in such cases
     C. Both
     D. Neither

139. Signs which may be present in the syndrome of pseudo-tumor cerebri include
     A. inferonasal field defects
     B. sixth nerve palsies
     C. both
     D. neither

140. Human magnesium deficiency results in
     A. tetany
     B. psychotic behavior
     C. both
     D. neither

141. Classic migraine
     A. usually improves during pregnancy
     B. is treated the same in pregnant and nonpregnant women
     C. both
     D. neither

142. Myasthenic features are associated with
     A. hypothyroidism
     B. hyperthyroidism
     C. both
     D. neither

143. Periodic paralysis is associated with
     A. hypothyroidism
     B. hyperthyroidism
     C. both
     D. neither

144. Cerebellar dysfunction is associated with
     A. hypothyroidism
     B. hyperthyroidism
     C. both
     D. neither

145. Myasthenia gravis is
    A. often exacerbated at the time of menstruation
    B. unaffected by birth control pills
    C. both
    D. neither

146. Known causes of pseudotumor cerebri include
    A. vitamin A excess
    B. nalidixic acid
    C. both
    D. neither

FOR EACH OF THE FOLLOWING QUESTIONS, ANSWER
(T)RUE OR (F)ALSE:

147. Oculoplethysmography and Doppler ultrasonography represent acceptable substitutes for arteriography in detecting carotid lesions.
    REF: Neurology 29:623, 1979

148. The Guillain-Barre syndrome is characterized by certain HLA types.
    REF: Ibid. , p. 743

149. With human axonal neuropathies, the CSF protein is usually markedly elevated.
    REF: Ibid. , p. 429

150. Diazepam is probably useful in halting the progression of dialysis encephalopathy.
    REF: Ibid. , p. 414

151. The typical patient with phenytoin-induced hepatotoxicity is black, female and has been taking the medication less than 6 weeks.
    REF: Ibid. , p. 177

152. Modified neurotoxin apparently does not prevent the progression of amyotrophic lateral sclerosis.
    REF: Ibid. , p. 77

153. Treatment of Huntington's disease with L-glutamate and pyridoxine for 2 years halted the progression of the disease.
    REF: Neurology 28:1281, 1978

154.   Follow-up of untreated patients with herpes simplex en-
       cephalitis discloses that over 90% are dead or vegetative.
       REF: Ibid. , p. 1193

155.   Lioresal in a double blind crossover study was not useful
       in treating the spasms of multiple sclerosis.
       REF: Ibid. , p. 1094

156.   Transient stuttering after stroke is associated with bi-
       lateral pathology.
       REF: Ibid. , p. 1159

157.   While CSF IgM is often elevated in multiple sclerosis, it
       bears no relation to the duration, severity or course of
       the disease.
       REF: Ibid. , p. 998

158.   Although one would expect the involuntary movements of
       Huntington's disease to improve with a cholinergic ago-
       nist, one, arecholine, made them worse.
       REF: Ibid. , p. 1061

159.   About 30% of multiple sclerosis patients are fully or par-
       tially employed 20 years after onset.
       REF: Neurology 28 (part 2):8, 1978

160.   The development of symptoms (none to maximum) in pa-
       tients with transient ischemic attacks usually takes 5-15
       minutes.
       REF: Stroke 9:299, 1978

161.   The usual duration of TIA's is 2-15 minutes.
       REF: Ibid.

162.   Stroke rehabilitation outcome is improved if the patient
       is placed in a rehabilitation center early.
       REF: Stroke 10:1, 1979

163.   In patients needing carotid surgery with a history of cor-
       onary artery disease, coronary artery bypass prior to
       or at the time of carotid surgery substantially reduces
       the postoperative survival.
       REF: Ibid. , p. 122

164.   Stroke is a less important cause of dementia than senile
       or presenile Alzheimer's disease.
       REF: Stroke 9:1, 1978

165. Fibromuscular dysplasia of the carotid arteries may be related to anticonvulsant drugs.
    REF: Ibid. , p. 172

166. Amaurosis fugax and hemispheric transient ischemic attacks differ considerably in their clinical and angiographic picture.
    REF: Ibid. , p. 254

167. Postoperative headache following carotid endarterectomy is uncommon.
    REF: Ibid. , p. 559

168. The most likely cause of the decline in stroke mortality in the United States is the decrease in adult cigarette smoking.
    REF: Ibid. , p. 549

169. Emergency carotid artery operation for stroke in evolution does more harm than good.
    REF: Ibid. , p. 599

170. Deficits from lacerations of the lower brachial plexus generally do not improve completely.
    REF: Mayo Clin. Proc. 53:803, 1978

171. Surgical exploration of brachial plexus injuries should be carried out in the face of clinical and myelographic evidence of root avulsion.
    REF: Ibid. , p. 805

172. Severe brachial plexus lesions resulting in a flail, anesthetic arm may best be served by shoulder arthrodesis, above elbow amputation, and a mechanical prosthesis with active rehabilitation.
    REF: Ibid. , p. 806

173. A close relationship exists between the severity of primary cerebral amyloid angiopathy and that of cerebral and visceral atherosclerosis.
    REF: Mayo Clin. Proc. 54:30, 1979

174. There is probably no need for a randomized study of external-internal carotid bypass surgery in patients with middle cerebral artery stenosis.
    REF: Ann. Neurol. 5:152, 1979

175. The localization of herpes simplex encephalitis to the temporal lobes is consistent with the existence of the latent virus in the trigeminal ganglia.
REF: Ibid., p. 2

176. Familial Creutzfeldt-Jakob disease is quite rare.
REF: Ibid., p. 177

177. Occipital lobe arteriovenous malformation and classic migraine are usually not distinguishable by clinical history.
REF: Ibid., p. 199

178. Blepharospasm has recently been successfully treated with clonazepam.
REF: Ibid., p. 401

179. Delayed visual evoked responses readily differentiate multiple sclerosis from pernicious anemia.
REF: Arch. Neurol. 36:168, 1979

180. There is a mild but definite decrease in intellectual performance of children with febrile seizures compared to their seizure-free siblings.
REF: Arch. Neurol. 35:17, 1978

181. Blood donations from descendants of familial Creutzfeldt-Jakob or Alzheimer's disease may pose a danger.
REF: Ibid., p. 697

182. Postinfectious encephalomyelitis may follow herpes simplex encephalitis treated with adenine arabinoside.
REF: N. Engl. J. Med. 300:1089, 1979.

183. True febrile convulsions are strongly associated with genetic factors.
REF: Epilepsia 18:495, 1977

184. Recurrent optic neuritis is not as significant as multiple lesions elsewhere in the nervous system in the establishment of the diagnosis of multiple sclerosis.
REF: Brain 101:495, 1978

185. The locked-in syndrome is most often due to a lesion confined to the basis pontis.
REF: Adams, R. D. and Victor, M.: Principles of Neurology, McGraw-Hill, New York, 1977, p. 196

186. The serum half-life of phenobarbital is usually much shorter than that of phenytoin.
REF: Ibid. , p. 227

187. Night terrors (pavor nocturnus) occur more often in children than in adults, during stage 3 or 4 sleep, and are not associated with an increased incidence of psychologic abnormalities.
REF: Ibid. , p. 249

188. Destruction of serotonergic neurons in the CNS results in decreased sleep.
REF: Ibid. , p. 245

189. Recurrent seizures more commonly follow thrombotic than embolic strokes.
REF: Ibid. , p. 526

190. Vasodilators (e. g. nicotinic acid, papaverine, etc.) are of proven benefit in stroke cases by increasing cerebral blood flow.
REF: Ibid. , p. 528

191. The margin between the dose of ethanol that produces surgical anesthesia and that which dangerously depresses respiration is wide.
REF: Ibid. , p. 776

192. Uremic encephalopathy is characterized by twitching and jerking, often leading to convulsions.
REF: Ibid. , p. 738

193. The pupillary light reflex is ordinarily retained in severe barbiturate intoxication.
REF: Ibid. , p. 794

194. "Charcot's triad" is a common combination of signs with which multiple sclerosis presents.
REF: Ibid. , p. 685

195. About 50% of multiple sclerosis patients relapse within 2 years.
REF: Ibid. , p. 684

196. Arteriosclerotic parkinsonism is clinically distinguished from the idiopathic form by its lack of tremor, lack of rigidity and lack of signs of bulbar palsy.
REF: Ibid. , p. 829

197.   Progressive supranuclear palsy is characterized by onset in a young adult with loss of reflex eye movements and retention of Bell's phenomenon.
         REF: Ibid. , p. 833

198.   The extraocular muscles and the sphincters are almost never involved in motor neuron disease.
         REF: Ibid. , pp. 842-843

199.   The incidence rate of amyotrophic lateral sclerosis of 1. 4 per 100, 000 is relatively constant for most countries.
         REF: Merritt, H. H. : A Textbook of Neurology, 6th ed. , Lea & Febiger, Philadelphia, 1979, p. 550

200.   With progressive supranuclear palsy downward gaze is affected first.
         REF: Ibid. , p. 518

201.   In Refsum's disease, cataracts are usually posterior subcapsular and they are seen in approximately 1/3 of the cases.
         REF: Dyck, P. J. , Thomas, P. K. , Lambert, E. H.: Peripheral Neuropathy, vol. II, W. B. Saunders Co. , Philadelphia, 1975, p. 870

202.   Carbamazepine (tegretol) commonly causes a severe leukopenia necessitating cessation of treatment.

203.   Amyotrophic lateral sclerosis occurs mainly in females and carries a worse prognosis if the onset is in the bulbar region.

204.   Propranolol in small doses (10-20 mg/day) is usually effective in the prevention of vascular headaches.

205.   A recently discovered diabetic came under complete control with diet, but some weeks later developed a footdrop. This is probably diabetic neuropathy.

206.   A swollen, tender scalp persisting for two days after a migraine is not unusual and needs no investigation.

207.   A severe mid-line vertex headache preceded by a binocular visual field loss and followed by confused behavior is consistent with basilar migraine.

208. Facial pain, hiccups and imbalance may each be the prominent symptom in the lateral medullary infarction syndrome.

209. Alcohol is probably a preferable remedy for essential tremor.

210. One should worry about nitrous oxide toxicity in dentists who show signs of spinal cord and peripheral nerve disease.

211. A patient has had a stroke with a right hemiparesis and mentions that his right eye was blind, too. This was most likely a hemianopsia.

212. You should suspect the diagnosis is incorrect if a myasthenic patient does not have extraocular muscle or lid weakness at the onset.

213. A patient with rampant muscle fasciculations also has moderate elevations of his serum CPK, therefore the diagnosis is unlikely to be ALS.

214. The Tensilon^R test used to determine further therapy in a very weak treated myasthenic may be misleading and the best thing to do may be to stop all medications and prepare to ventilate the patient for a few days.

215. A drink at night is probably the best thing for a patient with cluster headaches.

216. Carbamazepine should be stopped when the white blood cell count is below $4000/mm^3$.

217. Occult hydrocephalus may take months to become obvious.

218. Transient global amnesia may be precipitated by sexual intercourse.

219. "Giving way" is an unreliable sign of nonorganic weakness.

220. A sudden sharp stabbing pain behind the ear is usually not significant.

221. A 20-year-old lady is having trouble with intermittent numbness of her left little finger lasting an hour or two twice a week. This could be multiple sclerosis.

222. A factory worker with multiple sclerosis and mild upper motor neuron signs in the legs by exam, is denied disability on the basis of his nearly normal neurologic examination, but says his legs give out after he walks around for half an hour. These complaints can be organic, nevertheless.

223. A patient with mild diabetes, a tendency to alcoholism and a history of an old elbow fracture also has hypertrophic arthritis of his cervical spine. All four of these entities can present with symptoms of an ulnar neuropathy.

224. A patient with chronic parkinsonism is being treated with a combination of L-dopa and a dopa decarboxylase inhibitor, and gradually becomes severely demented and psychotic. The medication probably has nothing to do with his psychosis.

QUESTIONS 225 THROUGH 234 CONSIST OF NUMBERED ITEMS FOLLOWED BY LETTERED ITEMS. IN EACH CASE, MATCH THE NUMBERED ITEM WITH THE CORRECT LETTERED ITEM.

225. ___ Lepromatous leprosy

226. ___ Toxic neuropathy

227. ___ Subacute myeloopticoneuropathy

228. ___ Metabolic neuropathy

    A. Myxedema
    B. Treated with diaminodiphenylsulfone (dapsone)[R]
    C. Iodochlorhydroxyquin (Entero-Vioform[R])
    D. Lead, arsenic, thallium and organic mercury
    REF: Tower, Donald B., ed. in chief: The Nervous System, The Clinical Neurosciences, vol. 2, Raven Press, New York, 1975, p. 308

229. ___ Central sleep apnea

230. ___ Obstructive sleep apnea

231. ___ Mixed sleep apnea

    A. Bulbar poliomyelitis
    B. Myotonic muscular dystrophy
    C. High bilateral cervical cordotomy

232. ___ Sleep apnea syndrome

233. ___ Narcolepsy tetrad

234. ___ Monopolar depression

    A. Cataplexy
    B. Heavy snoring
    C. Psychomotor retardation

FOR THE FOLLOWING QUESTION, SELECT THE ONE MOST
APPROPRIATE ANSWER.

235. Medial cord injuries of the brachial plexus are clinically
similar to
  A. upper trunk lesions
  B. middle trunk lesions
  C. lower trunk lesions
REF: Mayo Clin. Proc. 53:802, 1978

FOR EACH OF THE FOLLOWING MULTIPLE CHOICE QUES-
TIONS, SELECT THE ONE MOST APPROPRIATE ANSWER:

236.   Which are characteristic of infant botulism?
        A. Extreme weakness with inability to suck or swallow
        B. Dilated fixed pupils
        C. Absent deep tendon reflexes
        D. All of these
        E. None of these
        REF: Pediatrics 59:321, 1977

237.   Fisher's syndrome
        A. consists of ataxia, external ophthalmoplegia and
            areflexia
        B. is felt by some to be an unusual form of Guillain-
            Barre syndrome
        C. is rare in children
        D. has a benign clinical course with complete recovery
        E. all of these
        REF: Ibid. , 60:726

238.   Melkersson-Rosenthal syndrome consists of
        A. recurrent facial paralysis with edema of lips
        B. edema of the hands and feet
        C. large smooth tongue
        D. hypertension
        E. all of these
        REF: Pediatrics 61:490, 1978

239.   Wilson's disease in children is best diagnosed by
        A. serum ceruloplasmin level
        B. increased urinary copper excretion
        C. abnormal liver function studies
        D. low serum copper levels
        E. liver biopsy for hepatic copper content
        REF: Ibid. , 62:47

240. Which of the following are characteristics of Reye's syndrome in infants under 6 months of age?
    A. Usually from rural areas
    B. Protracted vomiting common
    C. Usually from middle class homes
    D. Sudden onset of respiratory distress with apnea
    E. All of these
    REF: Ibid. , p. 84

241. Characteristics of familial dysautonomia in the first month of life include
    A. excessive sweating
    B. hypertonia
    C. small smooth tongue with absent fungiform papillae
    D. all of these
    E. none of these
    REF: Pediatrics 63:238, 1979

242. Phencyclidine (angel dust) intoxication is characterized by
    A. unresponsiveness
    B. vomiting and hypersalivation
    C. dystonic posturing
    D. generalized seizure activity
    E. all of these
    REF: J. of Pediatr. 94:316, 1979

243. Populations at increased risk for the development of future difficulties following the first febrile seizure include children
    A. whose first febrile seizure occurs at an early age (less than 18 months)
    B. who have complex febrile seizures
    C. who demonstrate abnormal neurological function
    D. who have a family history of afebrile seizures
    E. all of these
    REF: Ibid. , p. 177

244. Gelastic seizures
    A. may be defined as complex coordinated movements with grinning, giggling or joyful weeping
    B. are common in children
    C. in children are often caused by a tumor of the posterior hypothalamus
    D. A and C only
    E. A, B and C
    REF: Arch. Dis. Child. 53:965, 1978

245.   I-cell disease
         A. is an inherited disease
         B. clinically resembles Hurler's disease but without excessive urinary mucopolysaccharide excretion
         C. clinically and radiologically is apparent at birth
         D. is associated with severe mental retardation
         E. all of these
         REF: Arch. Dis. Child. 53:513, 1979

246.   The clinical features of seizure headaches include
         A. headache is usually diffuse or bifrontal
         B. headache may continue for hours but usually less than a day
         C. usually they are accompanied by nausea and vomiting and followed by a distinct postictal sleep
         D. usually they respond to anticonvulsants
         E. all of these
         REF: Dev. Med. Child. Neurol. 20:580, 1978

247.   Basilar skull fractures are present in children with head injury in
         A.   6-14%
         B.   20-25%
         C.   50%
         D.   30%
         E. none of these
         REF: Am. J. Dis. Child. 132:1121, 1978

248.   Recurrent headaches in children may represent migraine or seizure equivalents. Which of the following is true regarding these two diagnoses?
         A. Both respond equally well to DPH (diphenylhydantoin)
         B. DPH is more effective in the seizure equivalent group
         C. DPH is more effective in the migraine group
         D. The DPH response is dependent on the presence of EEG abnormalities
         E. None of these
         REF: Child's Brain 4:95, 1978

249.   Childhood aphasia
         A. occurs after left hemisphere lesion in 90-95% of cases
         B. is more likely to recover if the insult occurs before the age of 6 years
         C. tends to be predominantly nonfluent in kind
         D. studies indicate that crossed aphasia is no more frequent in children than in adults
         E. all of these
         REF: Ann. Neurol. 3:273, 1978

250. Bad prognostic factors for children with strokes include
   A. young age at the time of onset of hemiparesis
   B. onset with coma
   C. moyamoya syndrome
   D. A, B and C
   E. B and C only
   REF: Stroke 9:169, 1978

251. Which mucopolysaccharidosis is not transmitted in an autosomal recessive manner?
   A. Hurler
   B. Hunter
   C. San Filippo
   D. Scheie
   E. Maroteaux-Lamy
   REF: Farmer, T.W.: Pediatric Neurology, 2nd ed.,
   Harper & Row, Hagerstown, 1975, p. 180

252. Intelligence is usually normal in which mucopolysaccharidosis?
   A. Hunter
   B. San Filippo
   C. Hurler
   D. Scheie
   E. None of these
   REF: Ibid., p. 182

253. Which is not characteristic of infantile spasms?
   A. A common etiology is anoxia
   B. Onset after 1 year of age
   C. Often associated with tuberous sclerosis
   D. 90% of these children will be mildly or severely retarded
   E. 25% die within the first 3 years of life
   REF: Ibid., p. 49

254. The features of Refsum's disease include all of the folfowing except
   A. retinitis pigmentosa
   B. nerve deafness
   C. ataxia
   D. autosomal recessive transmission
   E. more common in black race
   REF: Ibid., p. 409

255. Which of the following reflexes found in the neonate and young infant may be elicited in children lacking cerebral hemispheres?
A. Sucking reflex
B. Grasp reflex
C. Moro reflex
D. Stepping reflex
E. All of these
REF: Ibid. , p. 28

256. Which of the following are characteristics of migraine headache in children?
A. Migraine begins before 16 years of age in less than 10% of cases
B. In girls the onset of migraine frequently coincides with the onset of menses
C. Cyclic vomiting is the dominant feature of migraine in small children
D. 2% of children develop symptoms of migraine during the first 10 years of life
E. B, C and D
REF: Ibid. , p. 70

257. Microphthalmia is frequently associated with
A. rubella syndrome
B. toxoplasmosis
C. trisomy 13-15
D. holotelencephalies
E. all of these
REF: Ibid. , p. 179

258. Narcolepsy
A. is common in early childhood
B. rarely appears during the teenage years or young adulthood
C. occurs in approximately half of the patients before the age of 10 years
D. characteristically features a rapid uncontrolled change of consciousness from a waking, alert state to sleep
E. all of these
REF: Swaiman, K. F. and Wright, F. S. : The Practice of Pediatric Neurology, C. V. Mosby Co. , St. Louis, 1975, p. 150

259.   A cherry red spot in the macula area may be seen with
       A.   Tay-Sachs disease
       B.   GM$_1$ gangliosidosis
       C.   Niemann-Pick disease
       D.   metachromatic leukodystrophy
       E.   all of these
       REF: Ibid. , p. 401

260.   The young infant does not develop hand preference until
       A.   18 months
       B.   6 months
       C.   12 months
       D.   7 months
       E.   none of these
       REF: Ibid. , p. 15

261.   Which reflex is not present at birth?
       A.   Moro
       B.   Palmar grasp
       C.   Landau
       D.   Rooting
       E.   Plantar grasp
       REF: Ibid. , p. 19

262.   Seizures in the newborn period are associated with
       A.   argininosuccinic aciduria
       B.   isovaleric acidemia
       C.   Joseph's syndrome
       D.   methylmalonic acidemia
       E.   all of these
       REF: Ibid. , pp. 360-394

263.   Which is not characteristic of phenylketonuria?
       A.   Blood phenylalanine level 20 mg/100 ml or higher
       B.   Urine positive for phenylpyruvic acid
       C.   Urine positive for 0-hydroxyphenylacetic acid
       D.   Tyrosine levels much higher than phenylalanine levels
       E.   Tyrosine levels low normal
       REF: Menkes, J. H. : Textbook of Child Neurology, Lea
       & Febiger, Philadelphia, 1974, p. 7

264. Maple syrup urine disease
      A. results from a defect in branched chain amino acid
          metabolism
      B. occurs only in the caucasian race
      C. is transmitted by an autosomal dominant gene
      D. results in structural alteration in the nervous system
          limited to cerebral gray matter
      E. all of these
      REF: Ibid. , p. 9

265. Myasthenia gravis in the child
      A. is more common in females
      B. usually occurs after 2 years of age
      C. is associated with poor response to medication and
          an irreversible course in 10-20%
      D. is associated with thyrotoxicosis in 10%
      E. all of these

266. Pyridoxine deficiency in early infancy is most often man-
      ifested by
      A. anemia
      B. hepatosplenomegaly
      C. seizures
      D. peripheral neuropathy
      E. respiratory distress

267. An infant should be transferring objects at
      A. 12 weeks
      B. 16 weeks
      C. 28 weeks
      D. 40 weeks
      E.   8 weeks

268. Hypocalcemia in the first 24-48 hours of life results from
      A. hypoxia
      B. prematurity
      C. maternal parathyroid disease
      D. all of these
      E. B and C only

269. The clinical features of holoprosencephaly include
      A. hypotelorism
      B. small head
      C. absence of nasal septum
      D. A and B
      E. A, B and C

270. The skin lesion most characteristic of neurofibromatosis
      is
      A. shagreen patch
      B. ash leaf lesion
      C. cafe-au-lait spot
      D. telangiectasia
      E. adenoma sebaceum

271. The area of the brain most often involved with herpes en-
      cephalitis is
      A. brain stem
      B. cerebellum
      C. temporal lobe
      D. occipital lobe
      E. none of these

272. Hydrocephalus is present in patients with myelomeningo-
      cele in the thoracolumbar region in
      A. 97%
      B. 80%
      C. 60%
      D. 90%
      E. 75%

273. The head circumference of a normal full term infant is
      A. 41 cm. $\pm$ 2
      B. 45 cm. $\pm$ 2
      C. 25 cm. $\pm$ 2
      D. 35 cm. $\pm$ 2
      E. 28 cm. $\pm$ 2

274. All the following are associated with an enlarging head,
      except
      A. hydrocephalus
      B. subdural hematoma
      C. Canavan's disease
      D. Krabbe's disease
      E. agenesis of the corpus callosum

275. Of the following, the condition least likely to cause sei-
      zures in the newborn period would be
      A. hypoxia
      B. intrauterine infection
      C. hypoglycemia
      D. intracranial hemorrhage
      E. congenital anomaly of the brain

276. Which cause of a floppy infant is not related to spinal cord involvement?
    A. Werdnig-Hoffmann disease
    B. Pompe's disease
    C. Tay-Sachs disease
    D. Cord injury
    E. Guillain-Barre

277. The following are characteristic of ataxia telangiectasia, except
    A. ataxia is clinically obvious by 4 years of age
    B. increased incidence of malignancy of the hematopoietic system
    C. recessive inheritance
    D. elevated IgE
    E. 50% of patients are moderately to markedly retarded

278. A one-year-old infant is brought to the hospital because of slow motor development. History reveals an early intolerance to milk, the development of jaundice and hepatomegaly. PE reveals a malnourished, retarded child with cataracts. The most likely diagnosis is
    A. mongolism
    B. phenylketonuria
    C. Hurler's syndrome
    D. galactosemia
    E. hypothyroidism

279. Galactosemia can be best diagnosed by
    A. PBI
    B. chromosome analysis
    C. increased mucopolysaccharides in urine
    D. serum phenylalanine level
    E. absent galactose -1- phosphate uridyl transferase

280. The average rate of growth of the head of a full term infant during the first six months of life is
    A. 0. 5 cm. /month
    B. 1. 5 cm. /month
    C. 1 inch/month
    D. 2. 5 cm. /month
    E. none of these

281. Which of the following diseases has both central white matter and peripheral nerve involvement?
    A. Schilder's disease
    B. Tuberous sclerosis
    C. Metachromatic leukodystrophy
    D. Periodic paralysis
    E. None of these

282. Which is not characteristic of subacute sclerosing panencephalitis?
    A. Elevated CSF protein
    B. Elevated CSF gamma globulin
    C. Suppression burst pattern on EEG
    D. Mental deterioration
    E. Elevated measles antibody titer in CSF

283. The lesion which is present in the newborn with tuberous sclerosis is
    A. adenoma sebaceum
    B. subungal fibroma
    C. ash leaf lesion
    D. localized gigantism
    E. all of these

284. A 4-year-old white male enters with a history of being increasingly unsteady with stumbling. His speech has become slower and he is excessively afraid. His reflexes are equal but hyperactive. His speech is slurred and he has body ataxia. The most likely diagnosis is
    A. behavior reaction
    B. porencephaly
    C. midline cerebellar tumor
    D. lesions from old skull fracture
    E. Schilder's disease

285. The most common cause of massive spasm is
    A. tuberous sclerosis
    B. brain tumor
    C. hypoxia
    D. neonatal meningitis
    E. head trauma

286. Sydenham's chorea is characterized by
    A. emotional instability
    B. muscle weakness
    C. purposeless, poorly controlled movements
    D. "Jack-in-box" tongue
    E. all of these

287. The diagnosis of reflex sympathetic dystrophy is based on findings which include
    A. dysesthesia
    B. edema
    C. hyperhidrosis
    D. extreme hyperesthesia
    E. all of these
    F. A, C and D only
    REF: J. of Pediatr. 93:84, 1978

288. Causes of acquired small heads (those infants who have a normal head circumference at birth but fail to have adequate head growth after birth) include
    A. hypoxia
    B. hypoglycemia
    C. polycythemia
    D. CNS infection
    E. all of these
    F. A and D only

QUESTIONS 289 THROUGH 307 CONSIST OF NUMBERED ITEMS FOLLOWED BY LETTERED ITEMS. IN EACH CASE, MATCH THE NUMBERED ITEM WITH THE CORRECT LETTERED ITEM.

289. ___ Tower of two blocks

290. ___ Rides a tricycle

291. ___ Pincer grasp

292. ___ Tower of 6 cubes

293. ___ Copies a circle

    A. 10 months
    B. 15 months
    C. 24 months
    D. 36 months

294. ___ Mandibulofacial dysostosis

295. ___ 21 Trisomy

296. ___ Riley bodies

297. ___ Micrognathia

298. ___ Broad thumbs

299. ___ XXY

300. ___ Rocker bottom feet

301. ___ XO

302. ___ Short arm 5th chromosome

     A. Turner's syndrome
     B. Hurler's syndrome
     C. Rubenstein-Taybi syndrome
     D. Pierre Robin syndrome
     E. Cri-du-chat syndrome
     F. Treacher-Collins syndrome
     G. Down's syndrome
     H. 13-15 trisomy
     I. Kleinfelter's syndrome

303. ___ Phenylketonuria

304. ___ Maple Syrup Disease

305. ___ Histidinemia

306. ___ Methylmalonic aciduria

307. ___ Tyrosinosis

     A. Purple ferric chloride reaction
     B. Green ferric chloride reaction
     C. Green-brown ferric chloride reaction
     D. Navy blue ferric chloride reaction
     E. Pale green ferric chloride reaction
     REF: Menkes, J.J.: Textbook of Child Neurology, Lea & Febiger, Philadelphia, 1974, p. 6

FOR EACH OF THE FOLLOWING QUESTIONS, ANSWER (T)RUE OR (F)ALSE.

308. Fibromuscular dysplasia should be considered in infants and children who develop acute hemiplegia.
REF: Pediatrics 59:899, 1977

309.   In a young mother (under 25 years of age) having one mongoloid child, the likelihood of a second afflicted infant is about 50 times greater than the random risk.
REF: Farmer, T. W. : <u>Pediatric Neurology</u>, 2nd ed. , Harper & Row, Hagerstown, <u>1975, p. 167</u>

310.   Menkes steely hair syndrome has been treated successfully with parenteral copper.
REF: <u>Arch. Dis. Child</u> 53:956, 1978

311.   Poor eyesight is one of the more common presenting complaints in homocystinuria.
REF: Ibid. , p. 242

312.   Lung volumes are reduced in infants who have intrauterine onset of Werdnig-Hoffmann disease.
REF: Ibid. , p. 921

313.   An intracranial bruit in an infant under the age of 4 months with symptoms of cardiac failure is strongly suggestive of a cerebral arteriovenous fistula.
REF: Ibid. , p. 592

314.   Intracranial bruits in children aged one to two are indicative of a focal lesion.
REF: Ibid.

315.   Brain malformations occur in 25% of infants with infantile spasms.
REF: <u>Epilepsia</u> 18:496, 1977

316.   Onset of the first seizure below 6 months of age is not significantly related to brain malformations, infantile spasms, or status epilepticus.
REF: Ibid. , p. 497

317.   Recent studies indicate that routine antibiotic prophylaxis in children with basilar skull fracture is unwarranted.
REF: <u>Am. J. Dis. Child.</u> 132:1121, 1978

318.   Extraneural metastases of medulloblastoma are sensitive to chemotherapy.
REF: Ibid. , p. 1004

319.   Concomitant chemotherapy with vincristine and methotrexate may potentiate the neurotoxic effects of CNS irradiation.
REF: <u>Ann. Neurol.</u> 4:47, 1978

320. Children with migraine respond equally well to anticonvulsants, analgesics and placebos.
REF: Neurology 29:506, 1979

321. Complete anosmia may be secondary to the Riley-Day syndrome (familial dysautonomia).
REF: Swaiman, K. F. and Wright, F. S.: The Practice of Pediatric Neurology, C. V. Mosby Co., St. Louis, 1975, p. 171

322. A child who has a second febrile seizure should be placed on daily anticonvulsants.

323. The one trisomy that is associated with a normal head circumference at birth is trisomy 21.

324. Less than 3 percent of patients who have rhabdomyomas of the heart have tuberous sclerosis.

325. The use of stimulant medication impairs cognitive functioning in 30% of children having symptoms of hyperactivity.
REF: Pediatrics 61:21, 1978

326. The absence of Kayser-Fleischer rings rules out Wilson's disease in the pediatric patient.
REF: Ibid., 62:47

327. Untreated patients with neurologic signs of Wilson's disease will always have Kayser-Fleischer rings.
REF: Ibid.

328. The majority of symptomatic pediatric patients with Wilson's disease respond to therapy with D-Penicillamine with normalization of hepatic, hematologic and neurologic function.
REF: Ibid.

329. The superior posterior part of the temporal lobe appears to be the cortical representation of the vestibular system.
REF: Pediatrics 59:833, 1977

330. Subacute necrotizing encephalomyelopathy or Leigh's syndrome has been associated with deficiency of cytochrome C oxidase in peripheral muscle.
REF: Ibid. 60:850

331. The administration of sodium benzoate has been successful in lowering the CSF glycine level to normal in patients with nonketotic hyperglycinemia.
REF: Pediatrics 63:369, 1979

332. The clinical course of acetaminophen overdose is often strikingly similar to Reye's syndrome.
REF: Pediatrics 61: 68, 1978

333. Altered valine metabolism has been reported to be responsible for the neurologic symptoms in a patient with an atypical form of maple syrup urine disease.
REF: Pediatrics 63:286, 1979

334. The term, hyperphenylalaninemic variants, is used to denote those children whose phenylalanine level is above 2 mg./dl. but below 20 mg./dl.
REF: Ibid., p. 334

335. Subacute sclerosing panencephalitis appears to occur as frequently following measles vaccination as following natural measles.
REF: Pediatrics 59:505, 1977

336. As a group, children with subacute sclerosing panencephalitis have measles at a later age than do age matched controls.
REF: Ibid.

337. Intracranial hemorrhage is more frequent in congenital factor VII deficiency than in classical hemophilia.
REF: J. of Pediatr. 94:413, 1979

338. Transcutaneous nerve stimulation has been unsuccessful in relieving the pain in reflex sympathetic dystrophy.
REF: J. of Pediatr. 93:84, 1978

339. Examination of a peripheral blood smear may suggest the diagnosis of infantile Pompe's disease.
REF: Ibid., p. 824

340. An increased risk of epilepsy is only minimal in children with febrile convulsions.
REF: J. of Pediatr. 94:177, 1979

341. The majority of recurrent febrile seizures will occur within 30 months of the onset of the disorder.
REF: Ibid.

342.   Oral glycine therapy may provide an approach to the man-
        agement of children with isovaleric acidemia which is
        superior to the dietary restriction of leucine.
        REF: J. of Pediatr. 92:813, 1978

343.   If seizures occur early after head injury, there is an 8%
        chance of recurrent late seizures during the first year
        after injury.
        REF: Farmer, T. W.: Pediatric Neurology, 2nd ed.,
        Harper & Row, Hagerstown, 1975, p. 46

344.   Recurrent convulsive seizures not associated with fever
        or systemic infection occur in 0.5% of children.
        REF: Ibid., p. 44

345.   Citrullinemia is a disorder of amino acid metabolism in-
        volving the urea cycle in which the primary defect appears
        to be a deficiency or absence of the enzyme argininosuc-
        cinic acid synthetase.
        REF: Ibid., p. 198

346.   Seizures are a prominent feature of phenylketonuria.
        REF: Ibid., p. 199

347.   The prominent clinical manifestation of Pelizaeus-
        Merzbacher disease consists of pendular oscillation of
        the globes in combination with titubation of the head.
        REF: Ibid., p. 210

348.   Akinetic seizures consist of sudden brief episodes of un-
        consciousness with no loss of postural tone.
        REF: Ibid., p. 49

IV: NEUROMUSCULAR DISORDERS

FOR EACH OF THE FOLLOWING MULTIPLE CHOICE QUES-
TIONS, SELECT THE ONE MOST APPROPRIATE ANSWER.

349. Subacute demyelinating polyneuropathy
     A. usually does not elevate the CSF protein
     B. may be recurrent
     C. responds equivocally to corticosteroid treatment
     D. all of these
     E. none of these
     REF: Arch. Neurol. 35:509, 1978

350. Overall, malignancy is seen in what percent of patients
     with polymyositis?
     A. 10-17%
     B. 20-30%
     C. 30-50%
     D. More than 50%
     E. None of these
     REF: Walton, J. N., ed.: Disorders of Voluntary Mus-
     cle, 3rd ed., Churchill Livingstone, Edinburgh, 1974,
     p. 616

351. Raynaud's phenomenon is seen in what fraction of patients
     with polymyositis?
     A. 1/4
     B. 1/3
     C. 2/3
     D. 3/4
     E. None of these
     REF: Ibid., p. 623

352. Myasthenia gravis involves
    A. 1/10, 000 to 1/50, 000 of the population
    B. females twice as often as males
    C. each sex with average onset at 20 years of age
    D. all of these
    E. none of these
    REF: Ibid. , p. 654

353. In cases of inherited sensory neuropathy type I, the most
    markedly decreased fibers on quantitative morphometric
    analysis are
    A. unmyelinated fibers
    B. large fibers
    C. large myelinated fibers
    D. B and C
    E. none of these
    REF: Dyck, P. J. , Thomas, P. K. , Lambert, E. H. :
    Peripheral Neuropathy, vol. II, W. B. Saunders Co. ,
    Philadelphia, 1975, p. 799

354. In cases of diabetic peripheral neuropathy
    A. there is ischemia of peripheral nerves
    B. there is accumulation of inhibitory substances inter-
       fering with normal Schwann cell activity
    C. osmotic changes occur due to accumulation of sugar
       alcohols (Sorbitol)
    D. all of these
    E. none of these
    REF: Ibid. , pp. 967, 972, 974

355. Which of the following neuropathies are due to parenchy-
    matous axonal degeneration?
    A. Acrylamide
    B. Porphyria
    C. Pernicious anemia
    D. All of these
    E. A and B only
    REF: Dyck, P. J. , Thomas, P. K. , Lambert, E. H. :
    Peripheral Neuropathy, vol. I, W. B. Saunders Co. ,
    Philadelphia, 1975, p. 332

356. Neonatal transient myasthenia gravis
    A. appears in infants born to mothers with myasthenia gravis
    B. usually lasts longer than 3 months
    C. appears to be related to the duration of the disease in the mother
    D. is prevented by performing thymectomy on the mother prior to pregnancy
    E. all of these
    REF: Farmer, T. W.: Pediatric Neurology, 2nd ed., Harper & Row, Hagerstown, 1975, p. 493

357. Neonatal persistent myasthenia gravis
    A. appears in infants born to mothers who do not have myasthenia gravis
    B. is characterized clinically by ptosis, external ophthalmoplegia and generalized weakness
    C. is not commonly associated with respiratory dysfunction
    D. is relatively resistant to drug therapy
    E. all of these
    REF: Ibid., p. 493

358. Nemaline myopathy is
    A. an essentially nonprogressive, proximal myopathy
    B. pathologically characterized by rod-like or thread-like structures without cross striations occupying the entire length of the involved muscle fiber
    C. characterized by proximal limb weakness with hypotonia, muscle wasting and diminished to absent deep tendon reflexes
    D. all of these
    E. none of these
    REF: Ibid., p. 499

359. In muscle carnitine palmityl transferase deficiency disease
    A. triglycerides are decreased
    B. cholesterol is markedly increased
    C. ketone bodies rise in plasma after the third to fourth day of fasting
    D. ketone bodies do not appear after an oral meal containing medium chain triglycerides
    E. none of these
    REF: Griggs, R. C., Moxley, T. T., eds.: Advances in Neurology, vol. 17, Treatment of Neuromuscular Diseases, Raven, New York, 1977, p. 134

360. Muscle stiffness after repeated intramuscular injection may be due to
A. Talwin (pentazocin)
B. repeated injection of normal saline
C. injection of antibiotics in adults
D. all of these
E. none of these
REF: Baker, A. B. and Baker, L. H. : Clinical Neurology, vol. 3, Harper & Row, Hagerstown, 1978, chapter 37, p. 56

361. Paramyotonia congenita is often associated with
A. bizarre high frequency potentials on EMG
B. no unusual sensitivity to cold
C. markedly hypertrophic muscles
D. paradoxical response to exercise
E. none of these

362. Facio-scapulo-humeral muscular dystrophy occurs
A. only in adults
B. only as an infantile form
C. primarily in females
D. in infants, adults, and as a late onset form
E. none of these

363. Neuromyotonia (Isaac's syndrome) is characterized by
A. muscle stiffness
B. increased sweating
C. myokymia
D. all of these
E. none of these

364. Patients with neuromyotonia respond well to
A. phenytoin
B. quinine
C. procainamide
D. all of these
E. none of these

365. Which of the following peripheral neuropathies is associated with marked autonomic dysfunction?
A. Diabetes
B. Alcoholic
C. Porphyria
D. Peroneal muscular atrophy
E. None of these

366.   Which test is most diagnostic of polymyositis?
        A. Electromyography
        B. Sedimentation rate
        C. Creatine phosphokinase
        D. Muscle histology and histochemistry
        E. None of these

367.   Marked improvement in motor nerve conduction veloci-
        ties is seen in patients with uremic neuropathy
        A. immediately following hemodialysis
        B. following peritoneal dialysis
        C. after renal transplantation
        D. all of these
        E. none of these

368.   Marked myoglobinuria occurs with
        A. type II glycogenosis (Pompe's disease)
        B. McArdle's disease
        C. carnitine myopathy
        D. all of these
        E. none of these

369.   Patients with carnitine palmityl transferase deficiency
        have
        A. markedly atrophic muscle
        B. fasciculations
        C. myoglobinuria following exercise
        D. all of these
        E. none of these

370.   Marked internal nuclei and ring fibers on muscle biopsy
        are seen predominantly in
        A. limb girdle or myotonic muscular dystrophy
        B. chronic neuropathy
        C. facio-scapulo-humeral muscular dystrophy
        D. all of these
        E. none of these

371.   Marked cardiac abnormalities occur in patients with
        A. limb girdle muscular dystrophy
        B. facio-scapulo-humeral muscular dystrophy
        C. myotonic muscular dystrophy
        D. all of these
        E. none of these

372.   The most acceptable proposed abnormality of myasthenia
        gravis is
        A. defective acetylcholine receptor protein at postsyn-
            aptic membrane
        B. abnormal quantum size at presynaptic level
        C. abnormalities in synaptic cleft
        D. all of these
        E. none of these

373.   The lesion in diabetic amyotrophy is
        A. degeneration of muscle tissue
        B. abnormalities in individual roots supplying the quad-
            riceps muscle
        C. neuropathy of femoral nerves
        D. all of these
        E. none of these

374.   Distal muscle weakness is characteristic of
        A. Duchenne's muscular dystrophy
        B. limb girdle muscular dystrophy
        C. myotonic dystrophy
        D. facio-scapulo-humeral muscular dystrophy
        E. all of these

375.   Pseudohypertrophy of muscle may occur in all the fol-
        lowing, except
        A. Duchenne's muscular dystrophy
        B. limb girdle muscular dystrophy
        C. facio-scapulo-humeral muscular dystrophy
        D. myotonic muscular dystrophy
        E. polymyositis

376.   Type I hereditary sensory neuropathy is inherited as
        A. dominant
        B. autosomal recessive
        C. sex-linked recessive
        D. none of these
        REF: Dyck, P. J. , Thomas, P. K. , Lambert, E. H. :
        Peripheral Neuropathy, vol. II, W. B. Saunders Co. ,
        Philadelphia, 1975, p. 795

377.   Which is the most common form of muscular dystrophy?
        A. Duchenne (pseudohypertrophic form)
        B. Limb girdle
        C. Facio-scapulo-humeral
        D. None of the above

378. The juvenile form of spinal muscular atrophy (Kugelberg-Welander disease) is inherited predominantly as
   A. sex-linked recessive
   B. autosomal dominant
   C. autosomal recessive
   D. none of these

379. Which disorder most commonly gives rise to mononeuritis multiplex?
   A. Connective tissue disease, i.e., lupus
   B. Trauma
   C. Leprosy
   D. Carcinomatous neuropathy

380. Which is the most acceptable explanation for sparing the pupillomotor fibers in diabetics?
   A. Due to central fascicular demyelination of the oculomotor nerve
   B. Lesion in the muscular branches of the nerve
   C. Due to primary muscle involvement
   D. None of these

381. Which neuropathy is most common world-wide?
   A. Alcoholic neuropathy
   B. Diabetic neuropathy
   C. Leprosy
   D. None of these

382. The inheritance of hereditary amyloid neuropathy is
   A. autosomal dominant
   B. autosomal recessive
   C. sex-linked recessive
   REF: Dyck, P.J., Thomas, P.K., Lambert, E.H.: Peripheral Neuropathy, vol. II, W.B. Saunders Co., Philadelphia, 1975, p. 1084

383. What is the effect of curarization on muscle abnormalities in cases of chondrodystrophic myotonia?
   A. Myotonia can be eliminated after nerve block by curarization
   B. Myotonia may increase after the nerve block by curarization
   C. The abnormalities are unchanged
   REF: Baker, A.B. and Baker, L.H.: Clinical Neurology, vol. 3, Harper & Row, Hagerstown, 1978, chapter 37, p. 49

FOR QUESTIONS 384-385, A STATEMENT IS FOLLOWED BY
FOUR POSSIBLE ANSWERS. ANSWER BY USING THE FOL-
LOWING KEY

    A. If only A is correct
    B. If only B is correct
    C. If both A and B are correct
    D. If neither A nor B are correct

384.   Myasthenia is associated with thymoma in 10% to 20% of
    cases.
    A. 60% of these patients are males
    B. This form of myasthenia usually appears at a later
        age
    C. Both
    D. Neither
    REF: Walton, J. N. , ed. : Disorders of Voluntary Mus-
    cle, 3rd ed. Churchill Livingstone, Edinburgh, 1974,
    p. 656

385.   Myotonia congenita is transmitted as
    A. autosomal dominant
    B. autosomal recessive
    C. both
    D. neither
    REF: Baker, A. B. and Baker, L. H. : Clinical Neurol-
    ogy, vol. 3, Harper & Row, Hagerstown, 1978, chapter
    37, p. 47

FOR EACH OF THE FOLLOWING QUESTIONS, ANSWER
(T)RUE OR (F)ALSE.

386.   Malignant hyperpyrexia should be added to cardiac con-
    duction defects, pulmonary insufficiency and untoward
    reactions to depolarizing agents as a potential anesthetic
    hazard for patients with well defined neuromuscular
    diseases.
    REF: J. of Pediatr. 93:83, 1978

387.   The peripheral neuropathy as measured by slowed motor
    conduction velocity in patients with myotonic dystrophy
    relates to their coexistent glucose intolerance.
    REF: Arch. Neurol. 35:741, 1978

388.   Females are affected with polymyositis twice as com-
    monly as males.
    REF: Walton, J. N. , ed. : Disorders of Voluntary Mus-
    cle, 3rd ed. , Churchill Livingstone, Edinburgh, 1974,
    p. 615

389. In polymyositis, upper extremity proximal muscles are affected before lower extremity muscles.
REF: Ibid. , p. 619

390. Abnormalities in serum protein and rheumatoid factor are seen in 50% of cases of polymyositis.
REF: Ibid. , p. 626

391. There is evidence that delayed hypersensitivity is an etiological factor responsible for polymyositis.
REF: Ibid. , p. 636

392. Polymyalgia rheumatica occurs mainly in late middle-aged males.
REF: Ibid. , p. 647

393. In myasthenia gravis with thymoma, muscle weakness is usually severe and difficult to control with anticholinesterase drugs.
REF: Ibid. , p. 656

394. In myasthenia gravis, flexor muscles in the upper extremities are more affected than extensor muscles.
REF: Ibid. , p. 657

395. About one in seven children born live to myasthenic mothers shows evidence of neonatal myasthenia.
REF: Ibid. , p. 663

396. Brachial plexus neuropathy is most common in adolescence.
REF: Dyck, P. J. , Thomas, P. K. , Lambert, E. H. : Peripheral Neuropathy, vol. I, W. B. Saunders Co. , Philadelphia, 1975, p. 664

397. In cases of carpal tunnel syndrome, the sensory conduction velocity may be normal even with sensory impairment.
REF: Ibid. , p. 694

398. Facio-scapulo-humeral muscular dystrophy is inherited in an autosomal dominant fashion.
REF: Dubowitz, V. and Brooke, M. H. : Muscle Biopsy: A Modern Approach, W. B. Saunders Co. , London, 1973, p. 202

399. A muscle concerned with precise movements may have a small number of muscle fibers per motor unit.

400. In clinical EMG, motor unit potential duration may vary with age.

401. Fibrillation potentials are seen exclusively in denervated muscle.

402. EMG findings in myopathy include increased numbers of polyphasic potentials and individual short duration motor unit potentials.

V: NEURO-OPHTHALMOLOGY

FOR EACH OF THE FOLLOWING MULTIPLE CHOICE QUES-
TIONS, SELECT THE ONE MOST APPROPRIATE ANSWER.

403.   Spontaneous pulsations of the retinal vein
        A. are present in 55% of unselected patients aged 20-90
        B. are related to blood pressure as a rule
        C. usually disappear at 190 mm. H_2O
        D. all of these
        E. none of these
        REF: Arch. Neurol. 35:37, 1978

404.   Pattern-shift visual evoked responses are
        A. abnormal in over 90% of persons with a history of
            optic neuritis
        B. normal in the absence of such a history
        C. specific for optic neuritis or multiple sclerosis
        D. all of these
        E. none of these
        REF: Ibid. , p. 65

405.   Forced downward ocular deviation is common with ocu-
        lovestibular testing in patients with
        A. head injuries
        B. mass lesions
        C. sedative drug-induced coma
        D. all of these
        E. none of these
        REF: Ibid. , p. 456

406. The blink reflex to light
    A. has an as yet unknown afferent pathway
    B. can be subcortically mediated
    C. may be preserved in neocortical death
    D. is not present with absent summated cortical visual evoked responses
    E. A, B and C
    REF: Arch Neurol. 36:53, 1979

407. Pathologic study of skew deviation has revealed lesions in the
    A. mesencephalon
    B. pons
    C. medulla
    D. B and C
    E. A, B and C
    REF: Arch. Neurol. 32:185, 1975

408. Herpes zoster ophthalmicus may cause dysfunction of the
    A. third cranial nerve
    B. sixth cranial nerve
    C. fourth cranial nerve
    D. all of these
    E. none of these
    REF: Arch. Ophthalmol. 96:1233, 1978

409. Hyaline bodies (Drusen) of the optic nerve head may be associated with which of the following characteristics?
    A. Disc appearance resembling papilledema
    B. Retinal hemorrhage
    C. Visual field loss
    D. All of these
    E. None of these
    REF: Arch. Ophthalmol. 97:65, 1979

410. In Osserman's classification of myasthenia gravis, Group I (ocular myasthenia) represents what proportion of the total?
    A. 5%
    B. 10%
    C. 20%
    D. 40%
    E. 60%
    REF: Ophthalmic Seminars 1:106, 1976

411. A 10-year-old girl presents with deficient abduction O. S.
      On examination, there is 40% limitation of abduction in
      the left eye. On attempted adduction, the palpebral fis-
      sure on the left narrows, with full ocular excursion and
      left enophthalmos. The diagnosis is
      A. left sixth nerve palsy
      B. thyroid eye disease
      C. Duane's syndrome
      D. myasthenia gravis
      E. none of the above
      REF: Ophthalmic Seminars 2:33, 1977

412. Visual evoked potential measurements in Parkinson's
      disease reveal
      A. normal latency
      B. prolonged latency
      C. decreased latency
      D. abnormal wave form
      E. A and D
      REF: Brain 101:661, 1978

413. Ophthalmoplegia, in cases of temporal arteritis, is due
      to
      A. extraocular muscle ischemia
      B. cranial nerve 3, 4 or 6 ischemia
      C. orbital swelling
      D. brainstem ischemia
      E. none of these
      REF: Brain 100:209, 1977

414. Structural mitochondrial abnormalities in chronic pro-
      gressive external ophthalmoplegia with ragged red fi-
      bers are present in
      A. liver cells
      B. somatic muscle
      C. neural tissue
      D. all of these
      E. none of these
      REF: Am. J. Ophthalmol. 83:362, 1977

415. Other causes of pupillary light-near dissociation besides
      Argyll-Robertson pupils include
      A. Adie's pupil
      B. aberrant regeneration of the third nerve
      C. diabetes mellitus
      D. all of these
      E. none of these
      REF: Surv. Ophthalmol. 19:290, 1975

416. Clinical findings in Horner's syndrome include
A. ptosis
B. miosis
C. "upside-down" ptosis
D. A and B
E. all of these
REF: Trans. Am. Acad. Ophthalmol. and Otol. 83:840, 1977

417. Sudden monocular visual loss in the sixth and seventh decades with an altitudinal field defect is characteristic of
A. optic neuritis
B. ischemic optic neuropathy
C. retrobulbar tumor
D. all of these
E. none of these
REF: Geriatrics 33:68, 1978

418. Progressive impairment of conjugate gaze may occur in
A. spinocerebellar degenerative disorders
B. Parkinson's disease
C. lipid storage disorders
D. all of these
E. none of these
REF: Ann. Neurol. 1:247, 1977

419. Opsoclonus
A. is a peculiar spontaneous involuntary ocular movement characterized by rapid, chaotic, conjugate eye movements of a multidirectional nature
B. is rarely continuous
C. does not occur when the eyes are closed
D. is diagnostic of Smith-Lemli-Opitz syndrome
E. all of these
REF: Dev. Med. Child Neurol. 19:57, 1977

420. A homonymous hemianopia with sparing of only the 60°-90° portion of the temporal hemifield indicates a/an
A. parietal lobe lesion
B. optic tract lesion
C. occipital lobe lesion
D. frontal lobe lesion
E. none of these
REF: Harrington, D. O.: The Visual Fields, C. V. Mosby Co., St. Louis, 1976, p. 332

421. Bilateral cecocentral scotomas have been reported secondary to
    A. ethyl alcohol
    B. lead
    C. digitalis
    D. all of these
    E. none of these
    REF: Ibid. , pp. 215-216

422. Bilateral severe concentric narrowing of the visual fields may be caused by
    A. hysteria or malingering
    B. retinitis pigmentosa
    C. bilateral occipital lobe infarcts
    D. all of these
    E. A and C only
    REF: Glaser, J. S. : Neuro-ophthalmology, Harper & Row, Hagerstown, 1978, p. 63

423. Rebound nystagmus is found in
    A. cerebellar disease
    B. cervical spine disease
    C. Meniere's disease
    D. normal populations
    E. all of these

424. Ocular bobbing is found in lesions of the
    A. cerebral hemispheres
    B. pons
    C. vestibular labyrinths
    D. thalamus
    E. all of these

425. Head nodding in spasmus nutans is
    A. compensatory, tending to offset the effects of the nystagmus
    B. noncompensatory, a result of the pathological process producing the nystagmus
    C. neither of these
    REF: Br. J. Ophthalmol. 60:652, 1976

426. Optic disc swelling in papilledema is due primarily to which of the following?
   A. Venous obstruction
   B. Interstitial compartment fluid accumulation
   C. Axonal swelling
   D. Glial swelling
   E. All of these
   F. None of these
   REF: Am. J. Ophthalmol. 83:424, 1976

427. Optic nerve field defects are characteristically
   A. cecal scotomas
   B. paracentral scotomas
   C. central scotomas
   D. none of these
   REF: Harrington, D. O.: The Visual Fields, C. V. Mosby Co., St. Louis, 1976, p. 231

428. In neuromyelitis optica, one-half of the cases show clinical onset of
   A. myelitis before optic nerve involvement
   B. myelitis and optic nerve involvement simultaneously
   C. optic nerve involvement before myelitis
   D. none of these
   REF: Ibid., p. 246

429. Cerebellar control over the vestibulo-ocular reflex is mediated via the
   A. vermis
   B. pyramis
   C. flocculus
   D. none of these
   REF: Brain Res. 40:81, 1972

430. See-saw nystagmus refers to a pattern of repetitive eye movements characterized by
   A. elevation and extorsion of one eye with depression and intorsion of the fellow eye
   B. elevation and intorsion of one eye with depression and extorsion of the fellow eye
   C. adduction and extorsion of one eye with depression and intorsion of the fellow eye
   D. none of these
   REF: Rose, F. C., ed.: Physiological Aspects of Clinical Neurology, Blackwell Scientific Publ., London, 1977, p. 23

QUESTIONS 431 THROUGH 433 CONSIST OF NUMBERED
ITEMS FOLLOWED BY LETTERED ITEMS. IN EACH CASE,
MATCH THE NUMBERED ITEM WITH THE CORRECT
LETTERED ITEM.

431. ___ Saccadic eye movements

432. ___ Smooth-pursuit movements

433. ___ Vestibular eye movements

    A. Involved in following a visual target; include the
       slow component of the opticokinetic response
    B. High-velocity movements involved in changing
       one's visual fixation from one object to another;
       include the fast component of vestibular and op-
       ticokinetic nystagmus
    C. Positional adjustment of the eyes in relation to
       the head
    REF: The Nervous System, Donald B. Tower, ed.
    in chief, vol. 2: The Clinical Neurosciences, Raven
    Press, New York, 1975, p. 481

FOR QUESTIONS 434-453, A STATEMENT IS FOLLOWED BY
FOUR POSSIBLE ANSWERS. ANSWER BY USING THE FOL-
LOWING KEY:

    A. If only A is correct
    B. If only B is correct
    C. If both A and B are correct
    D. If neither A nor B are correct

434. Bilateral failure of downward gaze may be associated
    with midbrain lesions medial and dorsal to the red nucleus
    A. unilaterally
    B. bilaterally
    C. both
    D. neither
    REF: Arch. Neurol. 35:22, 1978

435. Congenital oculomotor apraxia
    A. is characterized by normal voluntary horizontal gaze
    B. may be a disconnection syndrome
    C. both
    D. neither
    REF: Arch. Neurol. 36:29, 1979

436. Glissadic overshoots are due to
    A. pulse height errors
    B. pulse width errors
    C. both
    D. neither
    REF: Arch. Neurol. 35:138, 1978

437. Fluctuating ophthalmoplegia in the newborn may be caused
    by
    A. neonatal myasthenia
    B. metabolic abnormalities
    C. both
    D. neither
    REF: Neurology 27:971, 1977

438. Lower eyelid retraction is seen in
    A. Graves' disease
    B. central facial paresis
    C. both
    D. neither
    REF: Neurology 29:386, 1979

439. Botulism may cause
    A. progressive ophthalmoplegia
    B. miosis
    C. both
    D. neither
    REF: Arch. Ophthalmol. 95:1788, 1977

440. Patients with intracavernous aneurysms or meningiomas
    who have pupillary involvement may exhibit
    A. anisocoria
    B. isocoria
    C. both
    D. neither
    REF: Arch Ophthalmol. 96:457, 1978

441. Visual acuity in the newborn can be quantitated by
    A. flash visual evoked response
    B. optokinetic response to differential pattern grating
    C. both
    D. neither
    REF: Doc. Ophthalmol. 34:259, 1973

442. The following eye movement abnormalities have been reported in patients with hereditary cerebellar ataxia.
A. See-saw nystagmus
B. Cogwheel smooth pursuit
C. Both
D. Neither
REF: Brain 99:207, 1976

443. Oculomotor nerve paralysis alternating with spasm of the third nerve is seen with
A. congenital oculomotor nerve palsies
B. adult oculomotor nerve palsies
C. both
D. neither
REF: Surv. Ophthalmol. 20:81, 1975

444. Latent nystagmus is
A. congenital
B. acquired
C. both
D. neither
REF: Glaser, J. S., ed.: Neuro-ophthalmology, Harper & Row, Hagerstown, 1978, pp. 225-227

445. Photostress testing can be used to differentiate optic nerve disorders from
A. orbital disease
B. macular disease
C. both
D. neither
REF: Ibid., pp. 8-10

446. Colobomas of the optic disc may be associated with
A. basal encephalocele
B. pulsating exophthalmos
C. both
D. neither
REF: Ibid., pp. 74-76

447. Intra-orbital optic nerve sheath meningiomas may be associated with
A. disc swelling
B. optic atrophy
C. both
D. neither
REF: Ibid., pp. 120-121

448. Gaze-evoked nystagmus induced by tranquilizer or anti-
convulsant therapy commonly spares which gaze angle?
A. Upgaze
B. Down gaze
C. Both
D. Neither
REF: Ibid. , pp. 235-236

449. Incongruous homonymous hemianopias can be secondary
to lesions of the
A. optic tract
B. lateral geniculate body
C. both
D. neither
REF: Harrington, D. O. : The Visual Fields, C. V. Mosby
Co. , St. Louis, 1976, pp. 327-328

450. Periodic alternating nystagmus is usually associated with
lesions of
A. lower brain stem
B. upper brain stem
C. both
D. neither
REF: Rose, F. C. , ed. : Physiological Aspects of Clini-
cal Neurology, Blackwell Scientific Publ. , London, 1977,
p. 23

451. Cortical blindness may result from
A. generalized hypoxia
B. ictal phenomena
C. both
D. neither
REF: Glaser, J. S. and Smith, J. L. , eds. : Neuro-oph-
thalmology, Symposium of the University of Miami, C.
V. Mosby Co. , St. Louis, 1975, pp. 1-7

452. Eye signs in Graves' disease include
A. infrequent blinking
B. ptosis
C. both
D. neither
REF: Jones, I. S. and Jakobiec, F. A. : Diseases of the
Orbit, Harper & Row, Hagerstown, 1979, pp. 207-209

453. Inflammatory lesions of the orbit and orbital apex may be clinically associated with
    A. ophthalmoplegia
    B. Horner's syndrome
    C. both
    D. neither

FOR EACH OF THE FOLLOWING QUESTIONS, ANSWER (T)RUE OR (F)ALSE.

454. Unilateral papilledema in juvenile diabetics indicates a unilateral orbital or retro-orbital lesion.
    REF: Arch. Ophthalmol. 85:417, 1971

455. Experimental evidence indicates that hyperemia of the optic disc is an early sign of papilledema.
    REF: Arch. Ophthalmol. 95:1237, 1977

456. Enlargement of the blind spot is not seen in patients with pseudopapilledema and, thus, the field reliably differentiates true papilledema from pseudopapilledema
    REF: Arch. Ophthalmol. 97:71, 1979

457. Experimental evidence indicates that optic disc pallor results from decreased vascularity in the optic nerve head following axonal loss.
    REF: Ibid. , p. 532

458. Decline of visual function in patients with optic neuritis following exercise is commonly reported.
    REF: Br. J. Ophthalmol. 60:60, 1976

459. Surgical extirpation of intracanalicular meningiomas of the optic nerve sheath frequently improves vision.
    REF: Ophthalmology, 86:303, 1979

460. A unilateral lesion of the sixth nerve nucleus may clinically simulate an ipsilateral gaze palsy.
    REF: Brain Res. 112:162, 1976

461. Clinical evidence indicates that treatment of optic neuritis with ACTH favorably influences the final visual outcome.
    REF: J. Neurol. , Neurosurg. , Psychiat. 37:869, 1974

462. Isolated palsy of the inferior branch of the oculomotor nerve is frequently associated with posterior communicating aneurysms.
    REF: Ann. Neurol. 2:336, 1977

463. Oculomotor palsy from minor head trauma is a benign, though infrequent finding.
REF: J. A. M. A. 220:1083, 1972

464. Most patients with bilateral Adie's pupils have positive serological tests for syphilis.
REF: Trans. Am. Ophthalmol. Soc. 75:587, 1977

465. Optic atrophy associated with pituitary adenomas is a dependable preoperative indicator of poor postoperative visual return.
REF: Acta Ophthalmol. 55:208, 1977

466. Accommodative and pupillary abnormalities do not occur in myasthenia gravis.
REF: Br. J. Ophthalmol. 60:575, 1976

467. Orbital venography frequently is positive in patients with Tolosa-Hunt syndrome.
REF: J. Neurosurg. 44:544, 1976

468. Clinically noticeable anisocoria is present in 20% of the population at large.
REF: Glaser, J. S. , ed. : Neuro-ophthalmology, Harper & Row, Hagerstown, 1978, pp. 174-175

469. Optic gliomas of childhood are clinically similar to optic gliomas in the adult.
REF: Ibid. , pp. 116-120

470. Clinical characteristics of positional nystagmus induced by Nylen-Barany maneuvers frequently allow differentiation between a peripheral origin (end organ or nerve) and a central nervous system source.
REF: Ibid. , p. 235

471. Congenital nystagmus usually cannot be clinically differentiated from acquired forms of childhood nystagmus.
REF: Ibid. , p. 3

472. Optic nerve gliomas are most frequently present within the third and fourth decades.
REF: Jones, I. S. and Jakobiec, F. A. , eds. : Diseases of the Orbit, Harper & Row, Hagerstown, 1979, p. 417

473.   Tumor is a common cause of postganglionic Horner's
        syndrome.
        REF: Glaser, J. S. and Smith, J. L. , eds. : Neuro-oph-
        thalmology, Symposium of the University of Miami,
        C. V. Mosby Co. , St. Louis, 1975, pp. 265-269

474.   Contraction of the visual field is usually seen in stable
        or nonprogressive lesions.
        REF: Harrington, D. O. : The Visual Fields, C. V. Mosby
        Co. , St. Louis, 1976, pp. 107-111

475.   In ataxia telangiectasia, retinal telangiectasias are a
        constant feature of the syndrome.
        REF: Walsh, T. J. : Neuro-ophthalmology: Clinical
        Signs and Symptoms, Lea and Febiger, Philadelphia,
        1978, p. 129

476.   Oculopalatal myoclonus disappears during sleep.

477.   Vestibular nystagmus is more pronounced during concen-
        trated fixation.

478.   Pathologically, orbital pseudotumor and Tolosa-Hunt syn-
        drome are dissimilar processes.

FOR EACH OF THE FOLLOWING MULTIPLE CHOICE QUES-
TIONS, SELECT THE ONE MOST APPROPRIATE ANSWER.

479.   In patients with progressive supranuclear palsy, the EEG
        shows
        A.   marked increase in REM sleep
        B.   normal non-REM sleep patterns
        C.   patterns similar to those of patients with bilateral
             vascular lesions of the pons
        D.   all of these
        E.   none of these
        REF: Electroencephalogr. Clin. Neurophysiol. 45:16,
        1978

480.   In Reye's syndrome a somewhat specific EEG finding is
        A.   focal 3/sec. spike-wave bursts
        B.   diffuse slowing
        C.   phantom spike-waves
        D.   6 and 14/sec. positive spikes
        E.   none of these
        REF: EEG J. 40:645, 1976

481.   Occipital spikes during photic stimulation
        A.   are diagnostic of epilepsy
        B.   are seen only as part of the photoconvulsive response
        C.   are usually seen in posterior cerebral artery
             infarctions
        D.   correlate with visual field defects
        E.   none of these
        REF: EEG J. 39:93, 1975

482. A reversible isopotential EEG can occur in
    A. hepatic encephalopathy
    B. Reye's syndrome
    C. hyperthermia
    D. glioblastoma multiforme
    E. none of these
    REF: EEG J. 42:697, 1977

483. Alpha rhythm in a comatose patient implies
    A. full recovery
    B. probably recovery with neurologic deficit
    C. slight possibility of recovery
    D. permanent vegetative state
    E. certain imminent death
    REF: EEG J. 44:518, 1978

484. In brain abscesses, the EEG most commonly shows
    A. focal delta
    B. lateralized delta
    C. focal theta
    D. lateralized theta
    E. any of these
    REF: EEG J. 38:611, 1975

485. The alpha rhythm of the EEG
    A. is unrelated to age
    B. increases above age 60 as a rule
    C. is significantly correlated with head size
    D. is unrelated to head size
    E. B and D
    REF: Electroencephalogr. Clin. Neurophysiol. 44:344, 1978

486. The incidence of EEG abnormalities in the general psychiatric population is
    A. 0-25%
    B. 25-50%
    C. 50-75%
    D. 75-90%
    E. 90-100%
    REF: Clin. EEG 7:115, 1976

487. Appropriate reasons for obtaining an EEG in psychiatric patients include
    A. a history of seizures
    B. a family history of psychiatric disease
    C. the presence of psychosis rather than neurosis
    D. all of these
    E. A and B only
    REF: Ibid.

488. What is the significance of unilateral mu rhythm in the EEG?
    A. This is a normal finding
    B. This is a finding of no significance
    C. This implies contralateral disease
    D. This implies ipsilateral disease
    E. This is never seen as an isolated finding
    REF: Clin. EEG 9:181, 1978

489. What is the most common EEG abnormality in hydrocephalus?
    A. Diffuse theta
    B. Diffuse delta
    C. Spike-wave discharges
    D. Lateralized suppression
    E. Asynchronous sleep activity
    REF: Clin. EEG 6:29, 1975

490. In the differential diagnosis of intracranial hemorrhage, focal arrhythmic plus projected rhythmic delta favor
    A. intracerebral hematoma
    B. subdural hematoma
    C. epidural hematoma
    D. subarachnoid hemorrhage
    E. all of these
    REF: Clin. EEG 7:95, 1976

491. Which of the following substances tends to activate EEG seizure discharges?
    A. Milk
    B. Sugar
    C. Salt
    D. Alcohol
    E. None of these
    REF: Ibid. , p. 145

492. The EEG in rage attacks generally shows
A. anterior temporal spikes
B. 14 and 6/sec. spikes
C. mesial temporal sharp waves
D. diffuse temporal theta
E. no change
REF: Clin. EEG 9:131, 1978

493. The proper interpretation of 14 and 6/sec. spikes in the EEG is which of the following?
A. This is a normal finding of no significance
B. This is a form of seizure discharge
C. This is an abnormal finding with no clinical correlates
D. This finding is of uncertain significance but is associated with certain clinical conditions
E. None of these
REF: Clin. EEG 8:203, 1977

494. The EEG finding of PLED's (periodic lateralized epileptiform discharges) is most commonly seen in
A. vascular disease
B. tumor
C. encephalitis
D. epilepsy
E. multiple sclerosis
REF: Ibid., p. 191

495. 14 and 6/sec. positive spikes on the EEG are correlated with
A. headaches, dizziness, syncope, GI symptoms
B. syphilis
C. lupus erythematosus
D. ichthyosis
E. middle cerebral artery aneurysm
REF: Clin. EEG 9:52, 1978

496. Patients with PLED's (periodic lateralized epileptiform discharges) in their EEG are most commonly
A. alert
B. stuporous
C. confused
D. obtunded
E. comatose
REF: Clin. EEG 8:89, 1977

497. Which is incorrect regarding bilaterally recorded brain stem auditory evoked responses?
    A. Waves II to IV seem to originate in the central auditory pathway between the seventh nerve and the midbrain
    B. Wave V is specifically altered in midbrain lesions
    C. Wave I is specifically altered in supratentorial lesions
    D. Pontine lesions cause changes in waves II to IV
    E. Unilateral brain stem lesions can cause asymmetric alterations of the bilaterally recorded responses
    REF: Arch. Neurol. 36:161, 1979

498. In comatose patients with alpha rhythm in the EEG ("alpha coma"), cortical evoked potentials (EP) show the following pattern: (V=visual, A=auditory, SS=somatosensory).
    A. No EP's are seen
    B. V and A EP are present but not SS
    C. V EP are present but not SS or A
    D. SS and A are present but not V
    E. All EP's are present
    REF: Arch. Neurol. 32:713, 1975

499. In a patient with suspected seizures and a normal EEG, which follow-up procedure is most likely to disclose seizure activity?
    A. Repeat following prolonged sleep deprivation
    B. Repeat routine EEG
    C. Repeat with sphenoidal electrodes
    D. Repeat with nasopharyngeal electrodes
    E. No follow-up procedure is indicated since no seizure activity will be found
    REF: J. Neurol. 218:179, 1978

500. EEG changes related to a brain biopsy include
    A. focal spikes
    B. focal slowing
    C. focal increased amplitude and fast activity
    D. all of these
    E. none of these
    REF: J. Neurol. 211:95, 1975

501. The EEG changes in pernicious anemia correlate best with the
    A. degree of anemia
    B. amount of cerebral dysfunction
    C. serum B_{12} level
    D. degree of bone marrow change
    E. none of these
    REF: Mayo Clin. Proc. 51:281, 1976

502. An absence of EEG fast activity in epileptics given bar-
biturates indicates
A. patient noncompliance
B. toxic barbiturate levels
C. the need for another anticonvulsant
D. serious cerebral impairment from the epilepsy
E. A, B and D
REF: Eur. Neurol. 15:77, 1977

503. Following head trauma, accurate prediction of posttrau-
matic seizures can be made if the EEG
A. is normal
B. is diffusely slow
C. contains seizure discharges
D. contains focal slowing
E. none of these
REF: Eur. Neurol. 17:38, 1978

504. In what way may opening and closing the eyes be of diag-
nostic value during an EEG?
A. Midtemporal delta may be elicited
B. Triphasic waves may be suppressed
C. A seizure discharge may be precipitated
D. This never has any diagnostic value
E. None of these
REF: Electroencephalogr. Clin. Neurophysiol. 40:491,
1976.

505. What percent of patients with senile dementia have a nor-
mal EEG?
A. 0%
B. 20%
C. 40%
D. 60%
E. 80%
REF: J. Neurol. Neurosurg. Psychiat. 39:751, 1976

506. The EEG in cerebral arteritis most commonly shows
A. no change
B. focal slowing
C. focal seizure discharges
D. lateralized slowing
E. diffuse seizure discharges
REF: Child's Brain 4:1, 1978

507. The EEG in benign, noninfectious intracranial cystic disease (porencephaly, arachnoid cysts, etc.) in children is abnormal in
    A. 0-20%
    B. 20-40%
    C. 40-60%
    D. 60-80%
    E. 80-100%
    REF: Ibid. , p. 15

508. In childhood focal seizures, the most common EEG finding is
    A. diffuse spike-waves
    B. diffuse slowing
    C. focal slowing
    D. focal sharp waves
    E. none of these
    REF: Neuropaediatrie 8:3, 1977

509. In patients with complex partial seizures along with psychosis, the EEG is more likely to contain
    A. focal seizure discharges
    B. multifocal seizure discharges
    C. generalized seizure discharges
    D. slow waves
    E. all of these
    REF: Acta Neurol. Scand. 57:370, 1978

510. In alternating childhood hemiplegia, the EEG findings consist of
    A. no change
    B. diffuse slowing
    C. lateralized slowing which shifts with the hemiparesis
    D. slowing contralateral to the side of the initial hemiparesis
    E. diffuse beta
    REF: Arch. Dis. Child. 53:656, 1978

511. During the first week after head injury, the EEG in posttraumatic epilepsy shows seizure activity in
    A. 0-15%
    B. 25-50%
    C. 50-75%
    D. 75-90%
    E. over 90%
    REF: J. Oslo City Hosp. 27:89, 1977

512. A specific EEG finding permitting the impression of tumor is
A. focal delta
B. focal theta
C. focal delta decreasing rapidly with IV dexamethasone
D. diffuse delta
E. there is no way to be that specific in EEG interpretation
REF: J. Neurosurg. 48:601, 1978

513. Focal positive spikes and sharp waves in clinical EEG
A. are uncommon
B. are encountered chiefly in early life
C. suggest a search for simultaneous focal negative discharges
D. all of these
E. none of these
REF: Electroencephalogr. Clin. Neurophysiol. 42:15, 1977

514. The F-wave
A. estimates the fastest motor nerve conduction velocity
B. measures sensory nerve conduction velocity
C. is synonymous with H-reflex
D. is present only with upper motor neuron disorders
E. all of these
REF: Muscle and Nerve 1:181, 1978

515. Which of the following is the best predictor of subsequent neurologic status in neonates?
A. Apgar scores
B. Neurologic examinations
C. EEG
D. Fetal heart rate data
E. All are of equal value
REF: J. Pediatr. 90:985, 1977

516. Which of the following technical considerations must be taken into account in interpretation of an EEG showing electrocerebral silence?
A. What sensitivity settings were used
B. What filter settings were used
C. The recording time length
D. The use of a "noise" channel (2 electrodes on the hand)
E. All of these
REF: Am. EEG Soc., Guidelines in EEG, 1976

517. The EMG in the chondrodystrophic form of myotonia reveals
    A. typical myotonia
    B. spontaneous fibrillation
    C. myopathic features
    D. all of these
    E. none of these
    REF: Baker, A. B. and Baker, L. H.: Clinical Neurology, vol. 3, Harper & Row, Hagerstown, 1978, chapter 37, p. 49

518. Complete recovery from the state of electrocerebral silence (as properly defined) may occur in
    A. head trauma
    B. drug overdose
    C. hepatic encephalopathy
    D. epidural hematoma
    E. recovery never occurs
    REF: Baker, A. B. and Baker, L. H.: Clinical Neurology, vol. 1, Harper & Row, Hagerstown, 1978, chapter 12, p. 5

519. Chronic alcohol ingestion is likely to cause which of the following EEG changes?
    A. Excessive photic sensitivity
    B. Excessive buildup on hyperventilation
    C. 14 and 6/sec. positive spikes
    D. Small sharp spikes
    E. No change
    REF: Baker, A. B. and Baker, L. H.: Clinical Neurology, vol. 2, Harper & Row, Hagerstown, 1978, chapter 22, p. 6

520. Infantile spasms (Salaam attacks) are associated with
    A. 3/sec. spike and wave
    B. diffuse rhythmic fast spikes
    C. anterior temporal sharp waves
    D. multifocal spikes and slow waves
    E. all of these
    REF: Ibid., chapter 24, p. 17

521. The EEG in multiple sclerosis
    A. is diagnostic
    B. contains various abnormalities which are nondiagnostic
    C. shows focal delta in the area of the plaques
    D. usually shows seizure discharges
    E. is normal
    REF: Ibid., chapter 25, p. 35

522. Six months after a sudden left hemiparesis there is complete clinical resolution but persistent right EEG slowing remains. This is
A. part of the picture of a resolving CVA
B. indicative of a right hemisphere tumor
C. indicative of a right subdural hematoma
D. indicative of a right intracerebral hematoma
E. indicative of a recurrent CVA
REF: Baker, A. B. and Baker, L. H.: Clinical Neurology, vol. 1, Harper & Row, Hagerstown, 1978, chapter 3, p. 16

523. The EEG in the locked-in syndrome is characteristically
A. abnormal, showing electrocerebral silence
B. abnormal, showing diffuse delta
C. abnormal, showing suppression burst activity
D. abnormal, showing diffuse spike wave activity
E. normal or minimally abnormal
REF: Ibid., p. 18

524. In a child who suffers minor head trauma without loss of consciousness or neurologic abnormalities, the EEG shows diffuse delta with a focus contralateral to the area of trauma. What is the best interpretation of the EEG?
A. This is good evidence of a latent seizure problem
B. The child probably has a tumor
C. There is probably a meningitis secondary to the trauma
D. The findings can be secondary to the trauma
E. None of these
REF: Ibid., p. 25

525. In a patient with uremic encephalopathy, when the EEG shows diffuse delta, what clinical state can be expected?
A. Alert
B. Confused
C. Delirium
D. Coma
E. Clinical death
REF: Baker, A. B. and Baker, L. H.: Clinical Neurology, vol. 3, Harper & Row, Hagerstown, 1978, chapter 44, p. 2

526. EEG triphasic waves
   A. are diagnostic of hepatic encephalopathy
   B. while not diagnostic, occur in all cases of hepatic encephalopathy
   C. are nonspecific but limited to metabolic disease
   D. are nonspecific and occur in metabolic and nonmetabolic disease
   E. are normal
   REF: Ibid. , p. 7

527. The EEG in systemic lupus erythematosus may contain
   A. focal slowing
   B. diffuse slowing
   C. focal seizure discharges
   D. generalized seizure discharges
   E. all of these
   REF: Ibid. , p. 31

528. Abnormal EEG's in disorders of impulse control are seen in
   A. 0-25%
   B. 25-50%
   C. 50-75%
   D. 75-90%
   E. over 90%
   REF: Ibid. , chapter 46, p. 21

529. Nocturnal migraine attacks occur in
   A. stage 1 sleep
   B. stage 2 sleep
   C. stage 4 sleep
   D. REM sleep stage
   E. any stage
   REF: Baker, A. B. and Baker, L. H. : Clinical Neurology, vol. 2, Harper & Row, Hagerstown, 1978, chapter 13, p. 3

530. High doses of IV penicillin may cause which of the following EEG changes?
   A. Focal spikes
   B. Focal delta slowing
   C. Diffuse slowing
   D. Diffuse spike-wave discharges
   E. Sleep apnea
   REF: Ibid. , chapter 20, p. 43

531. In a patient with "rum fits" (alcohol withdrawal seizures)
      the EEG
      A. always shows focal seizure discharges
      B. often shows generalized seizure discharges
      C. shows seizure activity limited to the mesial temporal
          area
      D. shows diffuse slow waves
      E. is the same as in normal persons
      REF: Ibid. , chapter 22, p. 7

532. In coma secondary to head trauma, which is the most
      favorable EEG prognostic sign?
      A. Electrocerebral silence
      B. Suppression burst activity
      C. Sleep activity
      D. Alpha activity
      E. Low voltage delta activity
      REF: Gilroy, J. and Meyer, J. S. : Medical Neurology,
      2nd ed. , Macmillan Pub. Co. , New York, 1975, p. 466

533. The EEG in epidural hematoma with coma shows
      A. no change from normal
      B. ipsilateral slowing
      C. ipsilateral loss of faster frequencies
      D. diffuse slowing
      E. contralateral slowing
      REF: Ibid. , p. 473

534. In the diagnosis of infantile degenerative disease, an
      EEG finding suggesting gangliosiodoses is
      A. focal spikes
      B. paroxysmal theta
      C. irregular delta
      D. normal rhythms
      E. periodic complexes
      REF: Ibid. , p. 135

535. In the differential diagnosis of dementia, a low voltage
      EEG suggests
      A. Huntington's disease
      B. Alzheimer's disease
      C. Pick's disease
      D. Creutzfeldt-Jakob disease
      E. arteriosclerosis
      REF: Ibid. , p. 171

536. The cell membrane primarily has the electrical characteristics of a
    A. resistor
    B. transistor
    C. battery
    D. capacitor
    E. none of these
    REF: Aminoff, M. J. : EMG in Clinical Practice, Addison-Wesley Pub. Co. , Menlo Park, 1978, p. 13

537. EMG in Pompe's disease is characterized by
    A. diffuse fibrillation and positive sharp waves
    B. bizarre high frequency potentials resembling true myotonia
    C. marked polyphasics
    D. all of these
    E. none of these

538. Classical EMG findings in patients with periodic paralysis during the attack include
    A. complete electrical silence
    B. single unit interference pattern with short duration action potentials
    C. marked polyphasic activity
    D. B and C
    E. none of these

539. Which electromyographic abnormalities are seen characteristically in polymyositis?
    A. Combination of fibrillation potentials and polyphasics
    B. Marked fibrillation and positive sharp waves
    C. Pseudomyotonic discharges
    D. All of these
    E. None of these

540. Single fiber EMG is most helpful in which of the following conditions?
    A. Myasthenia gravis
    B. Limb girdle muscular dystrophy
    C. Peripheral neuropathy
    D. All of these
    E. None of these

541. Symmetrical rhythmic (regular, sinusoidal) slow EEG activity in a stuporous patient who is a known alcoholic is most suggestive of
   A. epidural hematoma
   B. head trauma
   C. acute drunkenness
   D. delirium tremens
   E. any of these

542. The presence of a normal EEG in an unresponsive patient suggests
   A. drug overdose
   B. hepatic encephalopathy
   C. diabetic coma
   D. ruptured basilar artery aneurysm
   E. none of these

543. What is the role of EEG nasopharyngeal electrodes in the diagnosis of temporal lobe epilepsy?
   A. Sharp activity from these electrodes should be carefully interpreted
   B. They are unnecessary in most cases
   C. Their use may obscure the diagnosis
   D. All of these
   E. None of these

544. Focal slow delta (1 H_Z or less) with adjacent normal rhythms in the EEG of a patient with a clinical picture of CNS infection is most consistent with
   A. meningitis
   B. brain abscess
   C. encephalitis
   D. brain tumor
   E. all of these

545. In a patient suspected of hypothyroidism the EEG is normal with alpha rhythm of 8 H_Z. What is the correct interpretation of this finding?
   A. Hypothyroidism is ruled out
   B. The diagnosis is confirmed
   C. There is no evidence supporting the diagnosis
   D. Although normal, the EEG findings may indicate early hypothyroidism
   E. None of these

546. The EEG findings in hepatic encephalopathy correlate
with
A. serum ammonia
B. total bilirubin
C. BSP abnormalities
D. the state of consciousness
E. none of these

547. Focal triphasic EEG waves are most suggestive of
A. hepatic encephalopathy
B. tumor
C. uremic encephalopathy
D. cerebral malaria
E. none of these

548. Periodic triphasic waves in the EEG of a 53-year-old
with dementia suggest
A. Creutzfeldt-Jakob disease
B. Alzheimer's disease
C. Pick's disease
D. Huntington's disease
E. arteriosclerosis

549. In multiple sclerosis, the sensory evoked potential un-
dergoes a relatively specific change consisting of
A. decreased amplitude of early wave components
B. increased latency of all wave components
C. loss of later wave components
D. a progressive increase of interwave latency
E. there is no specific change

550. Which statement applies to the role of sleep deprivation
in seizure evaluations?
A. A small percentage of patients will have seizure ac-
tivity not seen in natural or sedated sleep
B. This procedure may prohibit sleep recordings
C. Valuable data seen only in the waking EEG may be
lost
D. More than 24 hours of deprivation is required to see
an effect
E. All of these

551. Paroxysmal bursts of delta in the EEG of a suspected epileptic
    A. are as diagnostic as spikes or spike-waves
    B. confirm the diagnosis
    C. may represent abortive seizure discharges but must be considered nonspecific
    D. are considered normal
    E. none of these

552. Focal EEG slowing with adjacent spikes or sharp waves suggests
    A. a mass lesion
    B. middle cerebral artery thrombosis
    C. herpes encephalitis
    D. head trauma
    E. anoxic brain damage

553. Extremely periodic EEG bursts of sharp and slow activity in a child with dementia suggest
    A. Hallervorden-Spatz disease
    B. juvenile Huntington's disease
    C. metachromatic leukodystrophy
    D. Krabbe's disease
    E. SSPE

554. Focal left anterior temporal slowing in a 63-year-old male with headaches is
    A. normal
    B. indicative of a brain abscess
    C. indicative of hypertensive encephalopathy
    D. indicative of a middle cerebral artery thrombosis
    E. indicative of cerebral contusion

555. The EEG in Wallenberg's syndrome
    A. shows ipsilateral slowing
    B. shows contralateral slowing
    C. is normal
    D. shows diffuse slowing
    E. none of these

556. Periodic bursts of activity on an isopotential EEG background may signify
    A. status epilepticus
    B. suppression burst activity
    C. artefact
    D. all of these
    E. none of these

557. The EEG in narcolepsy
    A. may show sleep patterns during hyperventilation or photic stimulation
    B. often shows rapid eye movements within minutes after eye closure
    C. usually displays abnormal intrinsic cerebral activity in form and distribution
    D. A and B only
    E. all of these

558. Trace alternant in a premature infant is
    A. normal
    B. indicative of neonatal hypoxia
    C. indicative of neonatal birth trauma
    D. indicative of rupture of the vein of Galen
    E. indicative of H. Influenzae meningitis

559. EEG buildup (increased slowing and amplitude) lasts three minutes after hyperventilation in a 20-year-old with possible seizures. The correct interpretation is
    A. the finding confirms the diagnosis
    B. the finding is normal
    C. suggestive of mild hypoglycemia
    D. a nonspecific abnormality
    E. diagnostic of Moya-moya disease

560. Following removal of a low-grade astrocytoma from the right parietal area, the EEG shows right parietal delta plus sharp waves. Which of the following interpretations is correct?
    A. This is positive evidence of recurrence
    B. This is positive evidence of no recurrence
    C. There is probably a recurrence
    D. No statement regarding recurrence is possible
    E. None of these

561. Burr holes are made to drain a subdural hematoma. A postoperative EEG shows increased fast activity and increased amplitude over the burr holes. Which interpretation is correct?
    A. The EEG is normal
    B. The findings can be fully explained on the absence of bone
    C. The findings indicate some contusion associated with the hematoma
    D. The findings indicate rebleeding
    E. None of these

562. What is the clinical significance of EEG 6/sec. spike-wave activity (phantom spike-wave) in relation to epilepsy?
    A. This is a form of interictal seizure activity
    B. This is usually an ictal discharge associated with myoclonic jerks
    C. This is not a seizure discharge but is found more often in epileptics than the general population
    D. The finding has no clinical significance
    E. It is a normal finding

563. The clinical associations of 6/sec. spike-wave (phantom spike-wave) activity include
    A. drug ingestion
    B. headaches
    C. autonomic symptoms
    D. abdominal pains
    E. all of these

564. The relative localizing value of the EEG as compared to the somatosensory evoked potential (SSEP) in childhood hemiplegia is
    A. the SSEP is of more value
    B. the EEG is of more value
    C. both procedures localize equally well
    D. neither procedure is of localizing value
    REF: Dev. Med. Child Neurol. 18:620, 1976

565. Peroneal muscular atrophy may be divided into two types by electrophysiological techniques and nerve biopsy, characterized by
    A. demyelination or large axon loss
    B. normal biopsy or denervation EMG
    C. neurogenic and myogenic
    D. none of these
    REF: Brain 100:67, 1977

566. Which subcortical area has the lowest threshold for EEG seizures and overt convulsions following electrical stimulation?
    A. Insular cortex
    B. Amygdala
    C. Indusium grisium
    D. Hippocampus
    REF: Epilepsia 19:521, 1978

567. A diffusely slow EEG in the presence of abnormalities of serum calcium favors a diagnosis of
    A. hypocalcemia
    B. hypercalcemia
    C. either A or B
    D. neither A nor B
    REF: Baker, A. B. and Baker, L. H. : Clinical Neurology, vol. 3, Harper & Row, Hagerstown, 1978, chapter 43, p. 5

568. In treated cretinism, as compared with untreated, the EEG
    A. frequently converts from grossly abnormal to normal
    B. improves only slightly
    C. is equally abnormal in both conditions
    D. is normal in both conditions
    REF: Ibid. , p. 16

569. In hypoglycemia, the EEG, as compared to clinical signs and symptoms
    A. becomes abnormal but is less sensitive
    B. becomes abnormal but is more sensitive
    C. reflects lowered blood sugar levels as well as the clinical state
    D. is always normal
    REF: Ibid. , p. 26

570. The electrical potentials recorded from the human brain through the intact skull are of
    A. low amplitude, high frequency
    B. low amplitude, low frequency
    C. high amplitude, low frequency
    D. high amplitude, high frequency
    REF: Lenman, J. A. R. : Clinical Neurophysiology, Blackwell Scientific Pub. , Oxford, 1975, p. 263

571. Which of the following associations of alcohol and seizures is most common?
    A. Seizures related to alcohol withdrawal ("rum fits")
    B. Seizures secondary to uncomplicated head trauma
    C. Chronic seizures activated by alcohol and occurring later during abstinence
    D. Pre-existing seizures activated by alcohol ingestion
    REF: Gilroy, J. and Meyer, J. S. : Medical Neurology, 2nd ed. , Macmillan Pub. Co. , New York, 1975, p. 263

572. In patients with porphyria, electrographic alterations
A. tend to parallel the clinical state
B. include diffuse but not focal slowing
C. do not include focal spike-wave patterns
D. all of these
E. none of these
REF: Kooi, K. A. , Tucker, R. P. and Marshall, R. E.:
Fundamentals of Electroencephalography, 2nd ed. , Harper & Row, Hagerstown, 1978, p. 204

573. The EEG is normal in the face of a sudden aphasia and left hemiparesis. This indicates
A. a false-negative test
B. there is thrombosis of the basilar artery
C. the EEG is of no value in vascular accidents
D. the lesion is in the internal capsule

574. In a patient with an acute right middle cerebral artery thrombosis, the EEG shows right midtemporal delta as well as left-sided theta slowing. This means
A. there is diffuse vascular disease
B. the possibility of cerebral edema must be considered
C. there is another problem on the left
D. all of these

575. Newborn infants have peripheral nerve conduction velocities which are
A. 50% faster than adults
B. 25% slower than adults
C. 50% slower than adults
D. identical to adults

576. Cell membrane permeability to sodium ions is directly related to
A. voltage applied, i.e. membrane potential
B. sodium pump activity
C. potassium pump activity
D. none of these
REF: Aminoff, M. J. : EMG in Clinical Practice, Addison-Wesley Pub. Co. , Menlo Park, 1978, p. 14

FOR QUESTIONS 577-579, A STATEMENT IS FOLLOWED BY FOUR POSSIBLE ANSWERS. ANSWER BY USING THE FOLLOWING KEY:

    A. If only A is correct
    B. If only B is correct
    C. If both A and B are correct
    D. If neither A nor B are correct

577. An isoelectric EEG done by strict criteria, not associated with hypothermia, intoxication, or metabolic coma indicates
    A. irreversible brain death
    B. persistent vegetative state
    C. both
    D. neither
    REF: N. Engl. J. Med. 299:335, 1978

578. Motor nerve conduction velocities in patients with peroneal muscular atrophy have been shown to be
    A. markedly slow
    B. normal
    C. both
    D. neither
    REF: Aminoff, M. J. : EMG in Clinical Practice, Addison-Wesley Pub. Co. , Menlo Park, 1978, p. 5

579. Motor nerve conduction velocity is usually markedly slowed in
    A. axonal degeneration
    B. segmental demyelination
    C. both
    D. neither
    REF: Ibid.

QUESTIONS 580 THROUGH 582 CONSIST OF NUMBERED ITEMS FOLLOWED BY LETTERED ITEMS. IN EACH CASE, MATCH THE NUMBERED ITEM WITH THE CORRECT LETTERED ITEM.

580. ___ GM$_2$ Gangliosidosis (Tay-Sachs and Sandhoff's disease)

581. ___ Late infantile cerebromacular degeneration of Bielschowsky and Jansky (late infantile neuronal ceroid lipofuscinosis)

582. ___ Juvenile cerebromacular degeneration of Spielmeyer and Vogt (juvenile neuronal ceroid lipofuscinosis)

    A. No response to photic stimulation and no startle response

    B. Single high-amplitude polyphasic spikes biposteriorly with photic stimulation at low flash rates (less than 3 per second)

    C. Prominent startle response and no response to photic stimulation

    REF: Mayo Clin. Proc. 54:12, 1979

FOR EACH OF THE FOLLOWING QUESTIONS, ANSWER (T)RUE OR (F)ALSE.

583. Somatosensory evoked potentials show a reduced amplitude and prolonged latency in peripheral nerve diseases.
REF: Lenman, J. A. R. : Clinical Neurophysiology, Blackwell Scientific Pub. , Oxford, 1975, p. 278

584. A cerebral infarction often produces EEG changes similar to a tumor but this differentiation can be clarified by serial analysis.
REF: Ibid. , p. 281

585. A normal routine scalp EEG excludes significant cerebral disease.
REF: Ibid. , p. 283

586. In general, the threshold of excitability of a myelinated peripheral nerve fiber is directly proportional to the internodal spacing in that fiber, and thus to the size (diameter) of the fiber.
REF: Aminoff, M. J. : EMG in Clinical Practice, Addison-Wesley Pub. Co. , Menlo Park, 1978, p. 20

587. Myelinated peripheral nerve fibers conduct faster than unmyelinated ones because the local current circuits are confined to regions some distance ahead of the active region.
REF: Ibid. , p. 19

588. Conduction velocity in any peripheral nerve is directly related to the diameter of the axon.
REF: Ibid.

589.   The internal electrical resistance of peripheral nerve fibers is directly related to the fiber diameter.
REF: Ibid.

590.   The compound action potential recorded from a multifiber peripheral nerve represents the sum of the electrical events which occur in those of its fibers that are excited by the stimulus.
REF: Ibid.

591.   The major part of the cell membrane potential difference is generated by passive ionic movements (primarily the potassium ion).
REF: Ibid. , p. 12

592.   The saltatory conduction type of impulse propagation is seen in unmyelinated nerve fibers.

FOR EACH OF THE FOLLOWING MULTIPLE CHOICE QUES-
TIONS, SELECT THE ONE MOST APPROPRIATE ANSWER.

593. Which finding does not favor meningioma over acoustic
neuroma with a cerebellopontine angle mass demonstrated
on CT scan?
A. Increased attenuation
B. Marked calcification
C. Round shape
D. Center of tumor anterior to porus (internal acoustic
meatus)
E. Widening of porus
REF: Neuroradiology 17:22, 1978

594. A twenty-year-old man has had hemiparesis and seizures
since age 10 months. Skull films show dilated frontal sinus, elevated petrous ridge and thickening of the calvar-
ium, all on the right side only. Computerized tomography
reveals a dilated right lateral ventricle. The likely diagnosis is
A. cerebral hemiatrophy
B. Dyke-Davidoff syndrome
C. nonspecific brain insult in fetal or early childhood
development
D. all of these
E. none of these
REF: Ibid., p. 17

595. Scleral thickening with contrast enhancement on computerized tomography scan is a reliable sign for
    A. orbital pseudotumor
    B. thyroid eye disease
    C. optic nerve glioma
    D. meningioma of optic sheath
    E. all of these
    REF: Ibid. , 15:119

596. Which is the most helpful computerized tomography finding to distinguish Dandy-Walker syndrome from arachnoid cyst?
    A. Hypoplasia of the cerebellar vermis and hemispheres
    B. Elevation of the transverse sinus
    C. Obstructive hydrocephalus
    D. Demonstration of a CSF density midline cyst which does not displace the cerebellum
    E. None of these
    REF: Ibid. , p. 65

597. Which of the following is the least correct statement concerning complications of cerebral angiography?
    A. Serious neurologic complications are represented by new abnormal signs or symptoms or by aggravation of previously existing signs or symptoms
    B. The majority of complications related to cerebral angiography are transient
    C. Neurological complications may result from an embolus of thrombotic material outside or inside the catheter
    D. The most dangerous selective catheterization to perform in terms of highest complication rate is the right vertebral artery
    E. Complication rate for left vertebral catheterization is considerably greater than for carotid catheterization
    REF: Neuroradiology 14:175, 1977

598. Which is not a characteristic angiographic finding in patients with CNS lupus?
    A. Striking irregularities of contour of superficial and deep cerebral veins
    B. Stretching of subependymal veins indicating lateral ventricle enlargement
    C. Frequent arteriovenous malformations
    D. Diffuse aneurysmal changes
    E. Major cerebral artery occlusions
    REF: Ibid. , p. 59

599. Which statement is not true of computerized tomography and pneumoencephalography in patients with Huntington's chorea?
   A. Ratio of the distance between the two frontal horns and the intercaudate distance is decreased (1.33)
   B. The frontal horn/bicaudate ratio is significantly smaller than in normal patients
   C. This ratio statistically differentiates Huntington's chorea scans from those in patients with cerebral atrophy
   D. Pneumoencephalography is needed to clearly differentiate Huntington's from general cerebral atrophy
   E. Cortical atrophy is seen especially in the frontal areas
   REF: Ibid., 13:173

600. Which statement is not true regarding computerized tomography and radiation necrosis?
   A. It presents on CT scan as a mass lesion
   B. The lesion usually is seen as a region of abnormally diminished absorption
   C. The lesion enhances following contrast
   D. There is a relation of the intracerebral abnormality to the portals of previous irradiation
   E. It is easily distinguished from recurrent neoplasm
   REF: Neuroradiology 12:109, 1976

601. Which statement is not true of computerized tomography in patients with subarachnoid hemorrhage?
   A. Blood may be seen in the CSF cisterns for up to 5 days following hemorrhage
   B. A ruptured aneurysm can be localized by CT scan from the position of an intracerebral hematoma
   C. CT is less reliable than angiography in demonstrating multiple aneurysms
   D. CT is less reliable than angiography in determining which aneurysm bled when patient is found to have multiple aneurysms
   E. CT is less reliable than angiography in detecting arterial spasm
   REF: Neuroradiology 14:21, 1977

602. Which statement is **not** true regarding the differential diagnosis of suprasellar lesions?
    A. The most important criterion for differentiating basal meningiomas from other parasellar masses is the presence of hyperostosis whether demonstrated by computerized tomography or routine x-rays
    B. Craniopharyngiomas are much more frequently calcified than are pituitary adenomas
    C. Hydrocephalus is more frequent with pituitary adenoma than with craniopharyngioma
    D. Craniopharyngiomas will show contrast enhancement far less frequently than pituitary adenomas
    E. Aneurysms in the region usually present as eccentric round foci of increased absorption related to a portion of the circle of Willis
    REF: Radiology 120:95, 1976

603. Which statement is **not** true of computerized tomography for suprasellar masses?
    A. Portions of the suprasellar cistern may be demonstrated on routine CT in greater than 85% of cases
    B. Overlapping or thinner cuts demonstrate the anatomy of this region more frequently and clearly than the routine 13 mm slices
    C. At the usual scanning angle a slit-like third ventricle is normally seen in the midline between the flaring frontal horns and the quadrigeminal cistern
    D. When multiple cut CT is negative, pneumoencephalography is useful to show small lesions in this area
    E. When CT is positive, arteriography is required in some cases to rule out aneurysm prior to craniotomy
    REF: Ibid., p. 91

604. Which is the **least** common mass lesion seen in the suprasellar cistern on computerized tomography scan?
    A. Pituitary adenoma
    B. Hypothalamic glioma
    C. Meningioma
    D. Aneurysm
    E. Craniopharyngioma
    REF: Ibid.

605. Which statement is false concerning computerized tomography scans of patients with multiple sclerosis?
  A. Most patients with MS will have plaques that are demonstrable on CT
  B. Plaques seen on CT scan frequently do not correlate with the patient's signs and symptoms
  C. Ventricular dilatation appears to be compensatory for loss of white matter and the degree of dilatation is related to the number and size of plaques
  D. Acute MS lesions exhibit decreased or normal attenuation without contrast enhancement and increased attenuation with it
  E. The periventricular white matter is the most common location for MS plaques
  REF: Radiology 129:689, 1978

606. Which is not an advantage of Amipaque^R (Metrizamide) over Pantopaque^R for myelography?
  A. Not having to aspirate the contrast bolus at the end of the study
  B. Ability to demonstrate the subarachnoid spaces posterior to the conus medullaris and the upper cervical spinal cord
  C. Much lower incidence of arachnoiditis as a complication
  D. Much better visualization of the root sleeves in the lumbar region
  E. The cervical and lumbar areas may be evaluated during one examination
  REF: Ibid., p. 695

607. Which statement is least correct concerning metrizamide and/or radionuclide cisternography?
  A. Metrizamide and radionuclide cisternography correlate very closely in depicting CSF flow
  B. Transient ventricular reflux of metrizamide as indicated by the computerized tomography scan can occur in normal individuals
  C. Prolonged ventricular penetration (intraventricular metrizamide detectable at 48 hours or longer) is seen in patients thought to have communicating hydrocephalus
  D. In normal patients, metrizamide is visualized at 24 hours only in the parasagittal region
  E. Evaluation of flow over the convexities is shown better with metrizamide than with radionuclide cisternography
  REF: Radiology 130:681, 1979

608. Computerized tomography in a child with disseminated necrotizing leukoencephalopathy who has had previous radiation therapy to the brain reveals
   A. abnormal low density in the deep frontal cerebral white matter with areas of prominent calcification
   B. diffuse homogeneous areas of decreased density
   C. small lateral ventricles
   D. abnormal gray matter atrophy
   E. all of these
   REF: Radiology 130:371, 1979

609. Which is least correct concerning meningioma and skull bone patterns?
   A. Hyperostosis occurs in 25%-45% of cases
   B. Destructive or lytic changes occur in 10%-17% of cases
   C. Combined lytic and hyperostotic patterns occur
   D. Following surgery, tumors that presented with blastic changes recurred more frequently than those presenting with lysis (pure or mixed)
   E. Tumors that grow fastest tend to produce lytic changes while those that grow more slowly usually evoke blastic or hyperostotic change
   REF: Radiology 123:375, 1977

610. Which statement is not true of computerized tomography and acute head trauma?
   A. CT detects extracellular fluid as early as 3-5 hours following insult
   B. Peripheral contusions are clearly differentiated from extracerebral hematomas
   C. Cerebral edema may be the only pathologic finding following blunt head trauma
   D. Contusion appears on CT as multiple punctate blood-density foci within a prominent zone of edema
   E. Cerebral edema appears most intense 12-24 hours post injury
   REF: Ibid., p. 345

611. Which computerized tomography pattern is no longer present in patients six or more weeks after head trauma?
   A. Porencephaly
   B. Posttraumatic infarct (closed porencephaly)
   C. Communicating hydrocephalus
   D. Cerebral edema
   E. Subdural hematoma
   REF: Ibid.

612. Which statement is not correct concerning computerized tomography findings in children?
    A. The most common lesion producing enlargement of the optic nerve is a glioma
    B. The primary lesion to differentiate from optic nerve glioma is meningioma of the optic nerve sheath occurring in children with neurofibromatosis
    C. Capillary hemangioma frequently occurs in the orbit in infancy and usually involves the optic nerve
    D. Orbital rhabdomyosarcomas are very malignant lesions associated with bone destruction
    E. Retinoblastomas are usually calcified and enhance dramatically
    REF: Radiology 129:76, 1978

613. The computerized tomography detection rate for leptomeningeal spread of tumor is high in
    A. carcinoma
    B. lymphoma
    C. melanoma
    D. A and C only
    E. A, B and C
    REF: J. Comput. Assist. Tomogr. 2:448, 1978

614. Which statement about the optic nerve on computerized tomography is false?
    A. The optic nerve most frequently presents either a linear or slightly outward convex appearance
    B. The posterior intraorbital part of the optic nerve next to the optic canal is well visualized
    C. Increase in caliber and course tortuosity can be demonstrated in cases of papilledema
    D. Nystagmus may blur the optic nerve image
    E. Gaze shifts affect the course and CT appearance of the optic nerve
    REF: Ibid. , p. 141

615. Contralateral temporal horn widening seen on computerized tomography scan in patients with unilateral supratentorial mass lesions
    A. is a diagnostic sign indicating tentorial herniation
    B. occurs when tentorial herniation causes aqueductal compression
    C. often is associated with dilatation of the atrium and occipital horn as well on the side opposite the mass
    D. may be associated with shift of the brain stem with consequent widening of the angle cistern
    E. all of these
    REF: J. Comput. Assist. Tomogr. 1:319, 1977

616. Which is least correct concerning apparent cerebral atrophy on computerized tomography scan in patients on long-term steroids?
    A. The loss of brain volume in these patients is only due to steroid-induced protein catabolism
    B. Degrees of cerebral atrophy may be found that are not expected for the patient's age group
    C. There appears to be some correlation between dosage and degree of apparent atrophy
    D. There is surprisingly little clinical evidence of cerebral dysfunction associated with this apparent atrophy
    E. The appearance of the brain may improve following decrease or cessation of steroid use.
    REF: J. Comput. Assist. Tomogr. 2:16, 1978

617. Computerized tomography findings with cerebellar tumors usually do not include
    A. nonvisualization of the fourth ventricle
    B. displacement of the fourth ventricle
    C. normal-sized lateral ventricles
    D. obliteration or asymmetry of the quadrigeminal cistern
    E. narrowing of the pontine cistern
    REF: Semin. Roentgenol. 12:109, 1977

618. Which is not helpful in differentiating brain tumor and infarct?
    A. Presence of edema and mass effect on computerized tomography
    B. The clinical presentation
    C. Followup CT scan in 2-4 weeks
    D. Enhancement of lesion peripheral in the distribution of a major artery on CT scan
    E. Arteriography
    REF: Ibid., p. 107

619. Radionuclide brain scan may be superior to computerized two-dimensional tomography in
    A. greater accuracy in detecting intracranial lesions
    B. specific localization of lesions for planning surgical approach
    C. demonstration of edema
    D. diagnosing regions of hemorrhage
    E. detection of cystic or calcific areas in the lesion
    REF: Semin. Roentgenol 12:97, 1977

620. Which radiographic finding is <u>not</u> seen in neuro-fibromatosis?
   A. Enlargement of one or both optic foramina
   B. Enlargement or erosion of internal auditory canal
   C. Intraventricular tumor in atrium of lateral ventricle on computerized tomography scan
   D. Elevation of the lesser wing of the sphenoid and lateral displacement of the oblique orbital line
   E. A defect in the coronal suture
   REF: <u>Semin. Roentgenol.</u> 11:17, 1976

621. Which is <u>not</u> a cause of multiple intracranial calcifications?
   A. Healed brain abscesses
   B. Multiple sclerosis
   C. Neurofibromatosis
   D. Tuberous sclerosis
   E. Arteriovenous malformation
   REF: Ibid., p. 13

622. Computerized tomography evaluation is usually sufficient to avoid pneumoencephalographic investigation in which of the following?
   A. Chiari II malformation
   B. Proof of communication between porencephalic cavities
   C. Detecting intraventricular adhesions due to inflammatory processes
   D. All of these
   E. None of these
   REF: <u>J. Comput. Assist. Tomogr.</u> 1:204, 1977

623. The following entities may appear similar on computerized tomography scans. Which one is most likely to be differentiable from all of the others by its CT pattern?
   A. Alzheimer disease
   B. Generalized atrophy secondary to aging
   C. Chronic alcoholism
   D. Parkinsonism
   E. Multi-infarct dementia
   REF: <u>Semin. Roentgenol.</u> 12:63, 1977

624. Which is not a typical feature of Schilder's disease (diffuse cerebral sclerosis) detectable on computerized tomography scan?
    A. Widening of sulci
    B. Ventricular enlargement
    C. Propensity for frontal lobes
    D. Tendency to spread across corpus callosum
    E. Symmetry is rare early in the disease but may be present late in the course
    REF: Ibid., p. 70

625. Which is not true of cervicobasilar relationships?
    A. The basal angle is defined radiographically by the angle between two lines, the first drawn from the nasion to the tuberculum sella and the second drawn from the tuberculum to the anterior lip of the foramen magnum
    B. Platybasia (basal angle greater than 140 degrees) invariably accompanies basilar impression
    C. Chamberlain's line is drawn from the posterior edge of the hard palate to the posterior border of the foramen magnum
    D. Basilar impression is present when the odontoid tip extends more than 5 mm above Chamberlain's line
    E. A line connecting the mastoid tips is within 2 mm of the odontoid tip
    REF: Radiol. Clin. North Am. 15:155, 1977

626. Choose the one incorrect computerized tomography feature of acoustic neuromas.
    A. May be partially or nearly completely cystic
    B. Usually denser than surrounding brain on nonenhanced scan
    C. Sharply defined, densely blushing tumor masses on enhanced scan
    D. Confluent with the back of the petrous pyramid at the internal auditory canal
    E. May cause displacement of brain stem from the bone with widening of the basal cisterns
    REF: Norman, D., Korobkin, M., Newton, T. (eds.): Computed Tomography, C. V. Mosby Co., St. Louis, 1977, p. 231

627. Posterior fossa masses on computerized tomography scan cause
      A. distortion and displacement of the fourth ventricle
      B. widening or obliteration of the basal subarachnoid cisterns
      C. a variable degree of hydrocephalus
      D. zones of abnormal attenuation and abnormal contrast enhancement
      E. all of these
      REF: Ibid.

628. Which is not a feature of cerebellar astrocytomas on computerized tomography scan?
      A. May be cystic
      B. May be solid
      C. Some apparently well-defined lucent cystic tumors are found to be solid at surgery
      D. The cyst wall may blush after contrast but does not contain tumor cells when examined microscopically
      E. Some cystic tumors exhibit a mural nodule which blushes intensely after contrast
      REF: Ibid. , p. 234

629. In the early phases of cerebritis, computerized tomography scan
      A. may show no abnormality
      B. may show well-defined rim enhancement
      C. usually shows a low density mass which may have mottled areas of enhancement after contrast
      D. A and C only
      E. A, B and C
      REF: Ibid. , p. 319

630. Which is least correct regarding diagnosis of cerebral infarct on computerized tomography scan?
      A. Because of a low incidence of mass effect and a significant incidence of isodensity, the noncontrasted CT appearance of many infarcts will be normal
      B. The pattern of enhancement in cerebral infarction is characteristic for this disorder
      C. Between 7 and 28 days postinfarction, approximately two-thirds of cases will have demonstrable enhancement
      D. Areas of low density with unsharp margins are seen in most patients on noncontrasted CT during the first week postinfarction
      E. In confusing clinical situations with nonspecific initial CT scan, serial scans, radionuclide scan, or arteriography may be necessary to establish the diagnosis
      REF: Ibid. , p. 255

631. The "ring blush" at the site of a previous intracerebral hematoma, seen on computerized tomography
    A. indicates underlying neoplasm
    B. indicates supervening abscess
    C. appears localized to the periphery of the old hemorrhage
    D. disappears at two to six months after initial bleed
    E. C and D
    REF: Ibid. , p. 300

632. Choose the incorrect answer. The computerized tomography finding of a low density lesion with an enhancing rim
    A. is diagnostic of an abscess
    B. may be seen in gliomas
    C. may be seen in metastatic tumors
    D. can occur in resolving intracerebral hematomas
    E. can be seen in some infarcts
    REF: Ibid. , pp. 317, 320

633. Which statement is least correct concerning extracerebral hemorrhage on computerized tomography scan?
    A. Chronic subdural hematomas are of low density and characteristically have a biconvex shape
    B. Subdural hematomas usually extend over a far larger segment of the calvarium than epidural hematomas
    C. Recurrent acute subdural hematoma may be confined to the outer aspect of a chronic subdural hematoma producing extracerebral bands of different density
    D. The classic biconvex shape of the acute epidural hematoma can be mimicked by some acute subdural hematomas
    E. A very strong suggestive sign of an underlying iso-dense subdural hematoma is the presence of a thin, often faint curvilinear area of increased density at the interface of the brain and subdural collection
    REF: Ibid. , p. 303

634. The computerized tomography characteristics which favor a pyogenic abscess include
    A. a relatively thin rim with smooth inner margins following contrast enhancement
    B. multiloculation
    C. multiplicity
    D. all of these
    E. A and C only
    REF: Ibid. , p. 320

635.　Ventriculography is not useful in the investigation of which disorder of childhood?
A.　Raised intracranial pressure and presumed hydrocephalus, e. g. aqueductal stenosis
B.　Suspected Chiari malformation
C.　Suspected intraventricular tumor in presence of raised intracranial pressure
D.　Suspected congenital malformations of the brain
E.　As the initial procedure of choice for work-up of hydrocephalus
REF: Harwood-Nash, D. and Fitz, C. : Neuroradiology in Infants and Children, C. V. Mosby Co. , St. Louis, 1976, pp. 297-298

636.　When there is no clinical or radiologic evidence of raised intracranial pressure, a pneumoencephalogram is the definitive method of localization of the following tumors in children except
A.　mass lesions in and about the sella
B.　mass lesions in the cerebral hemispheres
C.　tumors about the posterior third ventricle
D.　brain stem gliomas
E.　tuberous sclerosis and concomitant small subependymal astrocytomas
REF: Ibid. , p. 227

637.　Cerebral angiography in children is least helpful for
A.　investigation of strokes
B.　suspected arteriovenous malformation
C.　suspected tumors
D.　suspected hydranencephaly
E.　differentiation of Dandy-Walker cysts from arachnoid cysts
REF: Ibid. , p. 318

638.　Which condition does not cause microcephaly?
A.　Mucopolysaccharidoses
B.　Intrauterine infection
C.　Hereditary micrencephaly of Penrose
D.　Neonatal cerebral ischemia
E.　Postmeningoencephalitis
REF: Ibid. , pp. 94-97

639. Which statement is incorrect regarding tumor circulation with meningiomas?
      A. Vessels within the tumor are usually regular except in angioblastic meningiomas
      B. Supply from meningeal vessels is diagnostic
      C. Tumor stain is uniform
      D. Tumor stain that persists into the venous phase is the most characteristic angiographic feature
      E. Early draining veins in the region of the tumor are sometimes seen
      REF: Newton, T. H. and Potts, D. G.: Radiology of the Skull and Brain, Angiography, Vol. II, Book 4, C. V. Mosby Co., St. Louis, 1974, p. 2268

640. Which statement is incorrect regarding early venous filling?
      A. It may be seen with glioblastomas
      B. It may occur with cerebral infarction
      C. It is the pathognomonic sign for arteriovenous malformation
      D. It may occur with inflammation including meningitis
      E. It may be noted with subdural empyema and cerebral abscess
      REF: Ibid., pp. 2506-2507

641. Which statement is not true with respect to epidural venography?
      A. The ascending lumbar vein on the symptomatic side is selectively catheterized if possible, but the contralateral vein may also be used successfully
      B. It is more difficult to interpret but equally accurate compared with myelography for diagnosis of herniated lumbar disc at L5-S1
      C. The extradural veins normally are symmetrical
      D. Unilateral or bilateral block of the anterior internal vertebral veins as they cross the interspace may be seen with disc herniation
      E. The anterior internal vertebral veins have a wavy pattern in frontal views because they course medially at the pedicles and then swing laterally at the disc spaces
      REF: Shapiro, R.: Myelography, 3rd ed., Year Book Pub., Chicago, 1975, pp. 566-583

642.   The myelographic finding of a clear-cut cap defect, cord
        displacement, and widened subarachnoid space on the
        side of the mass characterize which of the following?
        A. Herniated disc
        B. Metastatic disease
        C. Intradural, extramedullary lesion
        D. Extradural lesion
        E. Ependymoma
        REF: Ibid., pp. 143-144

643.   Which is not a tomographic finding indicative of patho-
        logic conditions involving the internal auditory canal?
        A. An enlargement of 2 mm or more in the measure-
            ment of one canal compared with the same point on
            the opposite canal
        B. Erosion of the posterior canal wall
        C. Disruption of the cortical white line surrounding the
            lumen of the canal
        D. Diameter of the internal auditory canal measuring
            10 mm
        E. Alteration in position of the crista falciformis from
            its normal position at or above the midpoint of the
            vertical diameter of the canal
        REF: Valvassori, G. E. and Buckingham, R. A.: Tomog-
        raphy and Cross Sections of the Ear, Thieme, Stuttgart,
        1975, p. 193

644.   Which is not true regarding postmeningitic hydrocephalus
        in infancy?
        A. Postmeningitic hydrocephalus in infancy may account
            for as many as 30% of all new cases of pediatric
            hydrocephalus
        B. Meningitis is less prone to cause CSF pathway block
            in infancy than later in life
        C. Fibrinous strands or thicker septa within the lateral
            ventricles may divide the ventricle into separate loc-
            uli and be seen on ventriculogram in a high percen-
            tage of cases
        D. CSF pathway obstruction is most frequent at the level
            of basal cisterns but may occur anywhere in the ven-
            tricular system
        REF: Neuroradiology 16:31, 1978

645. Which is not a feature of dural arteriovenous fistula of
the cavernous sinus?
A. Low flow, low pressure shunt
B. "Spontaneous" clinical onset
C. Arterial supply from meningohypophysial trunk on internal carotid injection
D. Does not have external carotid supply
REF: Ibid. , 15:41

646. The incidence of empty sella is not increased with
A. communicating hydrocephalus
B. hormone-producing pituitary tumors
C. chromophobe adenoma
D. increased intracranial pressure due to cerebral tumors
REF: Ibid. , 17:35

647. Which is not usually a feature of chronic subdural hematomas of infancy on computerized tomography?
A. Wide and prominent cerebral sulci
B. Large sylvian fissure
C. Effacement of lateral ventricles
D. Wide interhemispheric fissure
REF: Ibid. , 16:79

648. Medulloblastoma on computerized tomography scan typically does not show
A. intraventricular location
B. lucent halo around lesion
C. ring blush after contrast
D. homogeneous enhancement
REF: Neuroradiology 14:160, 1977

649. Present whole body computerized tomography scanners cannot demonstrate
A. the bony contour of the upper cervical canal
B. tonsillar herniation on scans done without intrathecal metrizamide
C. expanded cervical cord after intrathecal metrizamide
D. metrizamide entering a syrinx cavity
REF: Neuroradiology 15:73, 1978

650. Which is least correct concerning periventricular hypodensity on computerized tomography scan?
 A. Abnormal periventricular areas of decreased absorption (hypodensity) in the white matter are seen in a
variety of pathological conditions including hydrocephalus, multiple sclerosis, leukoencephalopathy,
viral inflammatory processes, and periventricular
spread of tumor
 B. The centrum semiovale is affected in leukoencephalopathy and spared in hydrocephalus
 C. The periventricular hypodensity in hydrocephalus
diminishes gradually from the ventricular wall toward
the cortex
 D. Density profiles are not helpful in distinguishing between white matter degeneration and hydrocephalus
 REF: Radiology 130:661, 1979

651. Myelographic features of spinal abscess in the subdural
space do not include
 A. bone changes of vertebral osteomyelitis adjacent to
myelographic block
 B. gradual transition zone with nodular defects project-
ing into the contrast column at the interface of the
block
 C. dorsal defect in the subarachnoid space placing the
lesion in extra-arachnoid location
 D. complete block at the level of disease
 REF: Am. J. Roentgenol. 132:138, 1979

652. Which statement is not true with respect to the great an-
terior medullary artery of Adamkiewicz?
 A. It arises from the left side of the aorta in 75% of
patients
 B. It originates between vertebral segments T9 and L2
in 85% of instances
 C. It is the principal arterial supply of the thoracolum-
bar cord
 D. It should not be selectively catheterized during
angiography
 REF: Shapiro, R.: Myelography, 3rd ed., Year Book
Pub., Chicago, 1975, pp. 257-263

653. Which is not true of tumor circulation in glioblastomas?
    A. Arteriovenous shunting is indicated by early drain-
       ing veins
    B. Drainage into deep central (deep medullary) veins is
       unusual
    C. It may be partially or completely avascular
    D. Bizarre, irregular tumor vessels are characteristic
    REF: Newton, T. H. and Potts, D. G.: Radiology of the
    Skull and Brain, Angiography, Vol. II, Book 4, C. V.
    Mosby Co., St. Louis, 1974, pp. 2275-2276

FOR THE FOLLOWING QUESTION, ANSWER (T)RUE OR
(F)ALSE.

654. Computerized axial tomography shows abnormalities in
    about 50% of patients with the Lennox-Gastaut syndrome
    and the most common abnormality demonstrated is dif-
    fuse cerebral atrophy.
    REF: Epilepsia 18:464, 1977

FOR EACH OF THE FOLLOWING MULTIPLE CHOICE QUES-
TIONS, SELECT THE ONE MOST APPROPRIATE ANSWER.

655.   Human toxic distal axonopathy is common with poisoning
       from all the following except
       A.   isoniazid
       B.   nitrofurantoin
       C.   mercury
       D.   disulfiram
       E.   N-hexane
       REF: Neurology 29:429, 1979

656.   The pathophysiology of myasthenia gravis is now thought
       to be
       A.   reduced numbers of acetylcholine quanta
       B.   reduced numbers of acetylcholine molecules per
            quanta
       C.   decreased number of acetylcholine receptors
       D.   hypersensitivity to acetylcholine
       E.   hyposensitivity to acetylcholine
       REF: N. Engl. J. Med. 298:136, 1978

657.   The afferent fibers stimulated by the noxious influence
       in the ciliospinal reflex
       A.   ascend to inhibit parasympathetic centers
       B.   do not cause pupillary changes without an intact
            brainstem
       C.   are necessary for the diagnosis of brain death
       D.   stimulate second order sympathetic neurons
       E.   A and B
       REF: Ibid. , 299:1314

658. The peak effect of amantadine in parkinsonism occurs
   A. in the first week
   B. at 6 months
   C. at one year
   D. at two years
   E. at three years
   REF: Ann. Neurol. 3:119, 1978

659. Patients with Huntington's disease have
   A. reduced gamma-aminobutyric acid levels in brain structures
   B. normal glutamic acid decarboxylase activity in brain
   C. normal CSF GABA
   D. all of these
   E. none of these
   REF: Arch. Neurol. 35:728, 1978

660. Which of the following drug categories can be related to increased EEG beta rhythm?
   A. Tricyclics
   B. Antihistamines
   C. Ethanol
   D. Benzodiazepines
   E. All of these
   REF: Clin. EEG 6:178, 1975

661. Which of the following neurotransmitters is believed to be involved in petit mal epilepsy?
   A. Aspartic acid
   B. Noradrenaline
   C. Gamma-aminobutyric acid (GABA)
   D. Serotonin
   E. None of these
   REF: Neuropharmacology 18:47, 1979

662. Which of the following are dopamine agonists (compounds which stimulate the synthesis or facilitate the action of dopamine)?
   A. Bromocriptine
   B. Levodopa
   C. Amphetamine
   D. All of these
   E. None of these
   REF: Can. J. Neurol. Sci. 6:87, 1979

663. Which of the following is suitable for the treatment of postanoxic intention myoclonus?
   A. Valproic acid
   B. 5-hydroxytryptophan
   C. Benzodiazepines
   D. All of these
   E. None of these
   REF: Ibid., p. 39

664. Parkinson's disease involves which of the following systems?
   A. Serotonergic enzymes
   B. Acetylcholinesterases
   C. Catecholamine enzymes
   D. All of these
   E. None of these
   REF: Ibid., p. 85

665. Anticonvulsants restore presynaptic inhibition by releasing
   A. excitatory neurohormone
   B. inhibitory neurotransmitters
   C. cyclic nucleotides
   D. high energy phosphate compounds
   E. none of these
   REF: Seeman, P. and Sellers, E. M.: Principles of Medical Pharmacology, University of Toronto Press, Toronto, 1976, pp. 264-265

666. Which is the key enzyme in the biosynthesis of catecholamines, dopamine, norepinephrine and adrenaline?
   A. Monoamine oxidase
   B. Catechol-o-methyl transferase
   C. Dopa decarboxylase
   D. Tyrosine hydroxylase
   E. None of these
   REF: Ibid., p. 231

667. The mechanism of action of the known alpha and beta adrenergic blockers (phenoxybenamine and propranolol) is
   A. blockade of endogenous transmitter at the postsynaptic receptor
   B. inhibition of enzymatic breakdown of transmitter
   C. blockade of transport system of axonal membrane
   D. all of these
   E. none of these
   REF: Ibid., p. 235

668. Cholinesterases are inhibited by organophosphate compounds in an irreversible fashion. However, they can be reactivated by specific agents, such as
   A. atropine
   B. PAM (pyridine-2-aldoxime)
   C. nicotine
   D. physostigmine
   E. all of these
   REF: Ibid., p. 205

669. Which condition is not an example of inborn errors of the urea cycle?
   A. Argininosuccinic aciduria
   B. Citrullinemia
   C. Congenital lysine intolerance
   D. Ornithine transcarbamylase deficiency with hyperammonemia
   E. Histidinemia
   REF: Menkes, J. H.: Textbook of Child Neurology, Lea & Febiger, Philadelphia, 1974, p. 15

670. Pompe's disease is
   A. glycogen storage disease type III
   B. the only type of glycogen storage disease that directly affects the central nervous system
   C. transmitted as a sex-linked recessive disorder
   D. characterized by the accumulation of glycogen in the skeletal muscles but not in the heart and liver
   E. all of these
   REF: Ibid., p. 28

671. The vascular supply to the spinal cord partly comes from the
   A. aorta
   B. subclavian arteries
   C. internal iliac arteries
   D. all of these
   E. A and B only
   REF: Adams, R. D. and Victor, M.: Principles of Neurology, McGraw-Hill, New York, 1977, p. 476

672. The blood transketolase assay is useful as an index of
   A. thiamine deficiency
   B. niacin deficiency
   C. ATP deficiency
   D. cyclic AMP deficiency
   E. none of these
   REF: Ibid., p. 752

673. Which condition is the result of abnormalities in lipid metabolism?
A. Gaucher's disease
B. Laurence-Moon-Biedl syndrome
C. Hurler's syndrome
D. Lesch-Nyhan syndrome
E. Lowe's syndrome
REF: Farmer, T. W.: Pediatric Neurology, 2nd ed.,
Harper & Row, Hagerstown, 1975, p. 208

674. Abetalipoproteinemia (Bassen-Kornzweig's disease) is the result of
A. defect of metabolism of exogenous phytanic acid
B. defect of intestinal and renal transport of neural alpha amino acids
C. defect of lipid-transporting peptides (apoLP-ser)
D. pyruvate decarboxylase deficiency
E. defect in serum immunoglobulin
REF: Ibid., p. 405

675. The majority of the optic tract receives its blood supply from the
A. anterior choroidal artery
B. posterior choroidal artery
C. posterior communicating artery
D. posterior cerebral artery
E. none of these
REF: Harrington, D. O.: The Visual Fields, C. V. Mosby Co., St. Louis, 1976, p. 91

676. Which is the basal ganglion disorder in which dopamine plays a major role?
A. Huntington's chorea
B. Wilson's disease
C. Hepatolenticular degeneration
D. Parkinsonism
E. None of these
REF: Siegel, G. J., Albers, R. W., Katzman, R. and Agranoff, B. W.: Basic Neurochemistry, 2nd ed., Little, Brown, 1976, p. 673

677. Which substance has been found to be abnormal in malignant hyperpyrexia?
    A. Increased calcium in the muscle sarcoplasmic reticulum
    B. Decreased potassium in the muscle sarcoplasmic reticulum
    C. Increased sodium in the muscle sarcoplasmic reticulum
    D. All of these
    E. None of these

678. Which of the following compounds can produce myotonia in humans?
    A. Clofibrate
    B. 20,25-diazocholesterol
    C. 2,4-dichlorophenoxyacetic acid
    D. All of these
    E. None of these

679. Neurologic complications of hypophosphatemia include
    A. mental obtundation
    B. weakness
    C. paresthesias
    D. all of these
    E. none of these

680. Magnesium intoxication results in a defect in
    A. cerebellar function
    B. neuromuscular transmission
    C. memory
    D. posterior column function
    E. all of these

681. The cerebral manifestations of eclampsia are
    A. usually secondary to hypermagnesemia
    B. secondary to an arteritis
    C. secondary to water intoxication
    D. sequelae of hypertension
    E. none of these

682. The following are manifestations of phenytoin hypersensitivity except
    A. erythema multiforme
    B. fulminant hepatitis
    C. Stevens-Johnson syndrome
    D. ataxia
    E. all of these

683.   Alcohol withdrawal seizures are enhanced by
        A.   reserpine
        B.   chlorpromazine
        C.   haloperidol
        D.   6-hydroxydopamine
        E.   all of these
        F.   none of these
        REF: Epilepsia 19:603, 1978

684.   There are many ways in which autonomic drugs can act.
        A drug may
        A.   mimic the normal transmitter
        B.   block the receptor occupied by the normal transmitter
        C.   cause the release of the normal transmitter from the
              nerve ending
        D.   interfere with storage or release of transmitters
        E.   all of these
        F.   B, C and D only
        REF: Seeman, P. and Sellers, E. M.: Principles of
        Medical Pharmacology, University of Toronto Press,
        Toronto, 1976, p. 230

685.   Entrapment of the anterior interosseous nerve has been
        reported to occur from
        A.   tendinous origin of the deep head of the pronator teres
        B.   tendinous origin of the flexor superficialis
        C.   accessory head of the flexor pollicis longus (Gantzer's
              muscle)
        D.   aberrant radial artery
        E.   all of these
        F.   A, B and C only

686.   In denervated organs, inhibition of acetylcholinesterase
        is without pharmacological effect.   The reason is
        A.   excess acetylcholine is accumulated
        B.   no acetylcholine is released
        C.   cholinesterase is abundant
        D.   none of these
        REF: Seeman, P., and Sellers, E. M.: Principles of
        Medical Pharmacology, University of Toronto Press,
        1976, p. 204

687.   L-dopa is converted to dopamine by
        A.   dopamine-beta-hydroxylase + ascorbic acid
        B.   monoamine oxidase + mitochondria
        C.   dopa decarboxylase + pyridoxal phosphate
        D.   none of these
        REF: Ibid., p. 231

688. The oxygen consumption by the brain in an adult young man weighing 70 kg. is about
    A. 5% of total body oxygen consumption
    B. less than 1% of total body oxygen consumption
    C. 20% of total body oxygen consumption
    D. insignificant as compared to total body consumption
    REF: Siegel, G. J., Albers, R. W., Katzman, R. and Agranoff, B. W.: Basic Neurochemistry, 2nd ed., Little, Brown, Boston, 1976, p. 394

689. Anomalies in the innervation of the hand muscles occur in
    A. less than 1% of persons
    B. 20% of persons
    C. 50% of persons
    D. over 50% of persons
    REF: Aminoff, M. J.: EMG in Clinical Practice, Addison-Wesley Pub. Co., Menlo Park, 1978, p. 145

690. Urinary copper excretion in Wilson's disease is
    A. increased
    B. decreased
    C. variable
    D. normal

691. The concentration of cyclic AMP in CSF of patients with motor neuron diseases is
    A. increased compared to controls
    B. decreased compared to controls
    C. unchanged
    REF: Andrews, J. M., Johnson, R. T. and Brazier, M. A. B.: Amyotrophic Lateral Sclerosis, Academic Press, Inc., New York, 1976, p. 109

FOR QUESTIONS 692-694, A STATEMENT IS FOLLOWED BY FOUR POSSIBLE ANSWERS. ANSWER BY USING THE FOLLOWING KEY.

    A. If only A is correct
    B. If only B is correct
    C. If both A and B are correct
    D. If neither A nor B are correct

692. In patients with Reye's syndrome, CSF monoamine metabolite levels show marked elevation of
    A. 5-hydroxyindoleacetic acid
    B. homovanillic acid
    C. both
    D. neither
    REF: Neurology 29:467, 1979

693. Sodium valproate
    A. hyperpolarizes the resting membrane potential due to an increase in membrane conductance to potassium
    B. causes increased whole-brain GABA levels
    C. both
    D. neither
    REF: Epilepsia 19:382, 1978

694. Acetylcholine is hydrolyzed in the body by
    A. pseudocholinesterase
    B. acetylcholinesterase
    C. both
    D. neither
    REF: Seeman, P. and Sellers, E. M.: Principles of Medical Pharmacology, University of Toronto Press, Toronto, 1976, p. 201

FOR EACH OF THE FOLLOWING QUESTIONS, ANSWER (T)RUE OR (F)ALSE.

695. Certain phenothiazines and butyrophenones also cause parkinsonism in man. Chlorpromazine produces this disorder by blocking the dopamine receptors in the CNS.
    REF: Cohen, M. M.: Biochemistry of Neural Disease, Harper & Row, Hagerstown, 1975, p. 169

696. The needs of the nervous system for high energy and rapid turnover are related to transmitter synthesis, release and uptake, to rapid conduction and ion pumping.
    REF: Gardner, E.: Fundamentals of Neurology, W. B. Saunders Co., Philadelphia, 1975, p. 99

697. Cerebral oxygen consumption is decreased during sleep.
    REF: Ibid.

698. The total lipid content is significantly decreased in white matter of Schilder's disease and subacute sclerosing panencephalitis patients compared to controls.
    REF: Siegel, G. J., Albers, R. W., Katzman, R. and Agranoff, B. W.: Basic Neurochemistry, Little, Brown, Boston, 1976, p. 584

699. The water content of white matter decreases in demyelinating disease due to the loss of myelin.
REF: Ibid. , p. 583

700. The pineal gland contains all the enzymes required for the synthesis of serotonin and two enzymes necessary for the subsequent use of the serotonin which are found in no other organ. The levels of serotonin in this gland are 50 times higher per gram than in whole brain.
REF: Cooper, J. R. , Bloom, F. E. and Roth, R. H. : The Biochemical Basis of Neuropharmacology, Oxford Univ. Press, New York, 1978, p. 203

701. Homovanillic acid and dihydroxyphenylacetic acid are the major metabolites of dopamine which are used as clinical indices.
REF: Ibid. , p. 172

702. Phenothiazine drug treatment causes a decrease in the levels of homovanillic acid and dihydroxyphenylacetic acid.
REF: Ibid.

703. Tyrosine is an important amino acid because it is the precursor for the synthesis of catecholamines.
REF: Ibid. , p. 122

704. The inhibitory neurotransmitter, gamma-aminobutyric acid, has been implicated in the pathogenesis of Huntington's disease, parkinsonism, epilepsy and schizophrenia.
REF: Ibid. , p. 224

705. The metabolism of diphenylhydantoin is inhibited by isoniazid to some degree in patients who are slow inactivators of isoniazid.
REF: Farmer, T. W. : Pediatric Neurology, 2nd ed. , Harper & Row, Hagerstown, 1975, p. 61

706. Patients with Refsum's disease have a defect in the alpha oxidation mechanism of beta methyl-substituted fatty acids.
REF: Dyck, P. J. , Thomas, P. K. and Lambert, E. H. : Peripheral Neuropathy, vol. II, W. B. Saunders Co. , Philadelphia, 1975, p. 875

707. Among the tricyclic antidepressants, the secondary amines are more effective for the treatment of depression with fewer side effects such as sedation and hypotension.
REF: Yamamura, H. I. , Enna, G. J. and Kuhar, M. J. : Neurotransmitter Receptor Binding, Raven Press, New York, 1978, p. 159

FOR QUESTION 708, A STATEMENT IS FOLLOWED BY FOUR POSSIBLE ANSWERS. ANSWER BY USING THE FOLLOWING KEY.

    A. If only A is correct
    B. If only B is correct
    C. If both A and B are correct
    D. If neither A nor B are correct

708. Acetylcholine actions resemble which of the following?
    A. Nicotine
    B. Muscarine
    C. Both
    D. Neither
REF: Seeman, P. and Sellers, E. M. : Principles of Medical Pharmacology, University of Toronto Press, Toronto, 1976, p. 202

QUESTIONS 709 THROUGH 719 CONSIST OF NUMBERED ITEMS FOLLOWED BY LETTERED ITEMS. IN EACH CASE, MATCH THE NUMBERED ITEM WITH THE CORRECT LETTERED ITEM.

709. ___ Hurler

710. ___ San Filippo A

711. ___ San Filippo B

712. ___ Scheie

713. ___ Maroteaux-Lamy

    A. Sulfatase B
    B. Alpha-acetylglucosaminidase
    C. Alpha-L-iduronidase (partial)
    D. Alpha-L-iduronidase
    E. Heparan sulfate sulfatase
REF: Menkes, J. H. : Textbook of Child Neurology, Lea & Febiger, Philadelphia, 1974, p. 32

714. ___ Dementia

715. ___ Barbiturate anesthesia

716. ___ Seizure activity

717. ___ Sleep (NREM)

718. ___ Halothane anesthesia

719. ___ Trichloroethylene anesthesia

A. Increase in cerebral blood flow
B. Increase in cerebral oxygen consumption plus increase in cerebral blood flow
C. Decrease in cerebral oxygen consumption plus decrease in cerebral blood flow
D. Decrease in cerebral oxygen consumption plus increase in cerebral blood flow
E. Decrease in cerebral oxygen consumption
REF: Lehman, J. A. R.: Clinical Neurophysiology, Blackwell Scientific Pub., Oxford, 1975, p. 18

FOR EACH OF THE FOLLOWING QUESTIONS, ANSWER (T)RUE OR (F)ALSE.

720. A reduction of the dose by 10 mg/kg/day is necessary for eliminating or preventing the hepatic side effects of valproate.
REF: Neurology 28:961, 1978

721. In some brain regions of patients with dominantly inherited olivopontocerebellar atrophy, the aspartic acid level is significantly lower than in controls.
REF: Neurology 27:257, 1977

722. The binding of valproic acid to human serum albumin is enhanced by phenytoin.
REF: Epilepsia 20:85, 1979

723. Free fatty acids significantly increase the valproic acid binding to human serum albumin.
REF: Ibid.

724. Sodium valproate, a widely used antiepileptic drug, is known to have a long biological half-life.
REF: Ibid., p. 61

725. Salivary concentrations of phenytoin and phenobarbital in patients receiving these drugs are equal to plasma concentrations.
REF: Ibid. , p. 37

726. There is an age-related decrease in beta-adrenergic receptors in human cerebellum.
REF: Life Sci. 24:367, 1979

727. Pharmacologic studies on myasthenic patients have, in general, indicated a postsynaptic disorder.
REF: Muscle and Nerve 1:153, 1978

728. The small amplitude miniature end plate potentials found in myasthenic patients are caused by a decrease in the number of reacting postsynaptic acetylcholine receptor sites.
REF: Ibid.

729. Calcium stimulated P-nitrophenylphosphatase and magnesium-dependent ATPase are elevated in erythrocyte membranes of patients with Duchenne and myotonic dystrophies.
REF: J. Neurol. Sci. 41:71, 1979

730. Vitamin E worsens some grand mal type seizures in man.
REF: Can. J. Neurol. Sci. 6:43, 1979

731. Acetylcholine probably is a synaptic transmitter of caudate nucleus interneurons.
REF: Brain 101:649, 1978

732. The absence of the glycine cleavage enzyme system in liver and brain accounts for the abnormally high glycine concentrations in the plasma and CSF of patients with nonketotic hyperglycinemia.
REF: Pediatrics 63:369, 1979

733. The pathogenesis of pancreatic encephalopathy is the action of released lipases and proteases from pancreatic enzymes.
REF: Adams, R. D. and Victor, M.: Principles of Neurology, McGraw-Hill, New York, 1977, p. 746

734. Cytotoxic edema is most commonly associated with brain tumor.
REF: Ibid. , p. 589

735. Acetylcholine has consistently been shown to be decreased in the basal ganglia of patients with Huntington's chorea.
REF: Ibid., p. 825

736. Tay-Sachs disease is a genetic disease also called GM_2 Gangliosidosis, type 2, which usually occurs in Jewish infants. The enzyme defect for this disease is lysosomal beta-D-N-acetylhexosaminidase.
REF: Cohen, M. M.: Biochemistry of Neural Disease, Harper & Row, Hagerstown, 1975, p. 107

FOR EACH OF THE FOLLOWING MULTIPLE CHOICE QUES-
TIONS, SELECT THE ONE MOST APPROPRIATE ANSWER.

737. The storage material which accumulates in metachroma-
tic leukodystrophy
A. is found principally in oligodendrocytes of cerebral
white matter
B. is a breakdown product of abnormal myelin
C. results from a deficiency of arylsulfatase A.
D. all of these
E. none of these
REF: Acta Neuropathol. 36:369, 1976

738. Microgyria results from a pathologic process operating
in the gestational period during the
A. 4th to 6th week
B. 3rd to 4th month
C. 5th to 7th month
D. 7th to 8th month
E. last month of pregnancy
REF: Ibid., p. 269

739. The pathogenesis of Cushing's disease has now been shown
to be most commonly
A. hypothalamic lesions
B. thalamic lesions
C. bilateral frontal lobe lesions
D. pituitary adenomas
E. none of these
REF: N. Engl. J. Med. 298:253, 1978

740. Select the most important single factor in the production of radiation myelopathy necrosis.
    A. High fraction size
    B. Shorter treatment time
    C. High total dose
    D. Increased length of cord treated
    E. None of these
    REF: Cancer 41:1751, 1978

741. Which of the following is not characteristic of ependymomas?
    A. Intracranial lesions are more common in children
    B. Intracranial lesions are more common than glioblastomas
    C. Intracranial lesions are mainly below the tentorium
    D. Intraspinal lesions are more common in adults
    E. Intraspinal lesions are most common in the cauda equina region
    REF: Cancer 40:907, 1977

742. The pathogenesis of central pontine myelinolysis is obscure. Which etiology seems least likely?
    A. Ischemia
    B. Nutritional and electrolytic imbalance
    C. Intoxication
    D. Lipolytic enzyme
    E. Hemorrhage
    REF: Pathol. Annu. 1:29-39, 1978

743. Sacrococcygeal teratomas are known to occur preferentially in
    A. full term infants
    B. females
    C. association with congenital anomalies
    D. all of these
    E. none of these
    REF: Arch. Pathol. Lab. Med. 102:420, 1978

744. The clinical manifestations of tuberous sclerosis appear during
    A. early infancy
    B. childhood
    C. adult life
    D. B and C only
    E. A, B and C
    REF: Ibid., p. 35

745. Hemorrhagic necrosis of cerebral white matter in infants is commonly associated with
A. sepsis
B. dehydration
C. cardiac disease
D. thrombosis of deep cerebral veins
E. all of these
REF: Ibid. , p. 40

746. Which is not characteristic of the cerebrohepatorenal syndrome of Zellweger?
A. Abnormal facies
B. Psychomotor retardation
C. Marked hypertonia
D. Failure to thrive
E. Early death
REF: Ibid. , p. 596

747. The pathological changes in Wernicke's encephalopathy and subacute necrotizing encephalomyelitis are similar. In SNEM, the lesions do not include
A. walls of the third ventricle
B. mammillary bodies
C. spinal cord
D. basal ganglia
E. cerebellum
REF: J. Neuropathol. Exp. Neurol. 36:128, 1977

748. Methyl mercury poisoning in utero causes
A. incomplete or abnormal migration of cortical and cerebellar neurons
B. derangement of cerebral and cerebellar organization
C. presence of heterotopic neurons, both isolated and in groups
D. all of these
E. none of these
REF: J. Neuropathol. Exp. Neurol. 37:719, 1978

749. Fibrinoid degeneration of intracerebral arterioles
A. is frequently associated with miliary aneurysms
B. is frequent in patients having malignant hypertension
C. may occur in nonhypertensive individuals
D. all of these
E. none of these
REF: Hum. Pathol. 8:133, 1977

750. Antibodies to acetylcholine play a role in the pathogenesis of myasthenia gravis because
    A. 87% of myasthenic patients have such antibodies
    B. they are bound to acetylcholine receptors
    C. the level of antibodies falls after thymectomy
    D. all of these
    E. none of these
    REF: Hum. Pathol. 9:495, 1978

751. The most common thymic lesion associated with myasthenia gravis is
    A. thymoma, benign
    B. thymic hyperplasia
    C. status thymolymphaticus
    D. thymoma, malignant
    E. none of these
    REF: Ibid.

752. Spinal arachnoiditis
    A. is about as common as intraspinal tumors
    B. is most common below the age of 20
    C. most commonly presents with nerve root pain
    D. pathologically, is a focal process in most cases
    E. A and C
    REF: Adams, R. D. and Victor, M.: Principles of Neurology, McGraw-Hill, New York, 1977, p. 474

753. Quantitative morphometric analysis in cases of Friedreich's ataxia shows which fibers to be predominantly decreased?
    A. Large myelinated fibers
    B. Small unmyelinated fibers
    C. Unmyelinated fibers
    D. B and C
    E. None of these
    REF: Dyck, P. J., Thomas, P. K. and Lambert, E. H.: Peripheral Neuropathy, vol. II, W. B. Saunders Co., Philadelphia, 1975, p. 819

754. The pathologic features of Menkes disease include
    A. cortical neuronal loss accompanied by gliosis
    B. myelin depletion
    C. predilection for neuronal loss in the hippocampus
    D. severe atrophy of the granular layer of the cerebellar cortex
    E. all of these
    REF: Dev. Med. Child Neurol. 20:586, 1978

755. A deficiency of peroxisomes is found in
    A. the cerebrohepatorenal syndrome
    B. the ataxia-telangiectasia syndrome
    C. Fabry's disease
    D. Pelizaeus-Merzbacher disease
    E. peroxide poisoning
    REF: Trump, B. F. and Jones, R. T. (eds.): Diagnostic Electron Microscopy, vol. 1, John Wiley and Sons, New York, 1978, p. 37

756. The neuropathy of addictive glue-sniffing (n-hexane toxicity)
    A. is largely a demyelination of large diameter axons
    B. is a giant axonal neuropathy
    C. is primarily a motor neuropathy
    D. has electrodiagnostic features of axon degeneration
    E. none of these
    REF: Asbury, A. K. and Johnson, P. C.: Pathology of Peripheral Nerve, W. B. Saunders Co., Philadelphia, 1978, p. 88

757. Which is not a typical feature of a metastatic intracerebral tumor?
    A. Calcifications
    B. Necrosis
    C. Endothelial proliferation
    D. Desmoplasia
    E. Discrete margins
    REF: Burger, P. C. and Vogel, F. S.: Surgical Pathology of the Nervous System and Its Coverings, John Wiley and Sons, New York, 1976, p. 355

758. Senescence related changes in dendritic architecture include
    A. proliferation of dendritic spines
    B. irregular swelling of neuron somata
    C. swelling of the initial segment of apical dendrites
    D. swelling at points of major dendrite bifurcation
    E. B, C and D
    REF: Res. Publ. Assoc. Res. Nerv. Ment. Dis. 57:107, 1979

759. Cerebral metastases of choriocarcinoma often present as
    A. intracerebral hematoma
    B. subarachnoid hemorrhage
    C. subdural hematoma
    D. cerebral arterial thrombosis
    E. all of these

760. The most common location for a supratentorial arach-
    noid cyst is
    A. parasagittal
    B. temporal lobe
    C. suprasellar
    D. frontal lobe
    E. occipital lobe

761. The most common location for an infratentorial arach-
    noid cyst is
    A. cerebellar hemisphere
    B. pons
    C. cerebellar tonsils
    D. midline cerebellar
    E. none of these

762. The characteristic clinical feature of status marmoratus
    is
    A. choreoathetosis
    B. spastic diplegia
    C. cerebral palsy
    D. spastic quadriplegia
    E. none of these

763. The most common intraspinal tumors are
    A. meningiomas and ependymomas
    B. ependymomas and sarcomas
    C. neurofibromas and sarcomas
    D. neurofibromas and meningiomas
    REF: Adams, R. D. and Victor, M.: Principles of Neu-
    rology, McGraw-Hill, New York, 1977, p. 489

764. Ragged red fibers
    A. is a term descriptive of the "moth-eaten" muscle fi-
       bers found in polymyositis and certain other
       myopathies
    B. are associated with decreased CSF immunoglobulins
    C. are typically found in the Kearns-Sayre syndrome
    D. result from abnormal collections of Z-band material
    REF: Brooke, M. K.: A Clinician's View of Neuromus-
    cular Disease, Williams and Wilkins, Baltimore, 1978,
    p. 168

765. In decreasing order of frequency, the most common primary sites of intracerebral metastatic tumors are
A. GI tract, lung, breast, pancreas
B. lung, breast, GI tract, prostate
C. breast, lung, GI tract, kidney
D. lung, breast, skin, kidney
REF: Burger, P. C. and Vogel, F. S.: Surgical Pathology of the Nervous System and Its Coverings, John Wiley and Sons, New York, 1976, p. 348

766. Almost pure axonal degeneration in peripheral nerves is produced by
A. acrylamide
B. lead
C. diphtheria toxin
D. triethyltin
REF: Asbury, A. K. and Johnson, P. C.: Pathology of Peripheral Nerve, W. B. Saunders Co., Philadelphia, 1978, p. 66

767. Spinal ventral nerve roots in Werdnig-Hoffmann disease show
A. atrophy of nerve fibers and astrocytic invasion
B. loss principally of nonmyelinated nerve fibers
C. focal demyelination with phagocytosis
D. no consistent histologic alterations until late in the disease
REF: Acta Neuropathol. 41:1, 1978

768. Whipple's disease
A. is a lipid storage disorder which frequently involves the CNS
B. may present with only CNS symptoms
C. is a reversible metabolic disorder
D. is caused by a virus
REF: Acta Neuropathol. 36:31, 1976

769. Wolman's disease is characterized by an accumulation of
A. neutral lipids in astrocytes, oligodendrocytes, and Schwann cells
B. myelin degradation products in CNS macrophages
C. cholesterol in oligodendrocytes
D. none of these
REF: Acta Neuropathol. 45:37, 1979

770. Tangier disease of adult onset has striking resemblance to syringomyelia with several common characteristics except
    A. wasting of intrinsic hand muscles
    B. impairment of cutaneous pain and temperature sensations
    C. chronic course
    D. neuropathic and lipid abnormalities
    REF: J. Neuropathol. Exp. Neurol. 37:138, 1978

771. Medullo-epitheliomas exhibit which of the following characteristics?
    A. They are rare neoplasms
    B. They are highly malignant
    C. They occur in early childhood
    D. They are common in the cerebrum
    E. All of these
    F. None of these
    REF: J. Neuropathol. Exp. Neurol. 36:712, 1977

772. Neurofibrillary tangles are found in
    A. Guam parkinsonism dementia complex
    B. postencephalitic parkinsonism in neurons of the substantia nigra
    C. the cortex of adult Down's syndrome
    D. the cortex of dementia pugilistica
    E. all of these
    F. A, B and C only
    REF: Res. Publ. Assoc. Res. in Nerve. Ment. Dis. 57:99, 1979

FOR QUESTIONS 773-778, A STATEMENT IS FOLLOWED BY FOUR POSSIBLE ANSWERS. ANSWER BY USING THE FOLLOWING KEY.

    A. If only A is correct
    B. If only B is correct
    C. If both A and B are correct
    D. If neither A nor B are correct

773. The severity of prognosis in sacrococcygeal teratomas depends on the presence of which of the following structures within the teratoma?
    A. Yolk tumor sac elements
    B. Neuroectodermal components
    C. Both
    D. Neither
    REF: Arch. Pathol. Lab. Med. 102:420, 1977

774. A characteristic histopathological and ultrastructural feature in mannosidosis is a generalized ballooning of nerve cells containing vacuoles filled with
A. mannose-rich oligosaccharide granules
B. glycogen granules
C. both
D. neither
REF: J. Neuropathol. Exp. Neurol. 36:807, 1977

775. Cerebral hemorrhagic infarction may result from perfusion of blood through ischemic areas in
A. a retrograde manner through collateral channels
B. an anterograde manner via reopening of vascular channels
C. both
D. neither
REF: Ibid., p. 338

776. The mononuclear cells responding to injury in the central nervous system are of
A. local origin
B. hematogenous origin
C. both
D. neither
REF: Ibid., p. 74

777. Asphyxia in the developing brain may cause
A. damage to polyribosomes
B. impairment of protein synthesis
C. both
D. neither
REF: J. Neuropathol. Exp. Neurol. 37:85, 1978

778. Hypertrophy of the pyramidal tract is
A. a rare condition
B. associated with infantile hemiplegia
C. both
D. neither
REF: Ibid., p. 34

FOR EACH OF THE FOLLOWING QUESTIONS, ANSWER (T)RUE OR (F)ALSE.

779. Delayed postanoxic encephalopathy is often characterized pathologically by demyelination.
REF: Adams, R. D. and Victor, M.: Principles of Neurology, McGraw-Hill, New York, 1977, p. 734

780. The striking pathologic change in hepatic encephalopathy
is necrosis and degeneration of neurons.
REF: Ibid. , p. 737

781. The most common site of origin of oligodendrogliomas
is in the frontal lobes.
REF: Ibid. , p. 597

782. Chordomas most commonly occur in the thoracic area
of the spinal cord.
REF: Ibid. , p. 611

783. Lymphomas and astrocytomas are the most common tumors at the foramen magnum.
REF: Ibid. , p. 614

784. Histologically, the characteristics of Schilder's disease
are in marked contrast to those of multiple sclerosis.
REF: Ibid. , p. 690

785. Spinal leptomeningeal metastases from a primary intracranial glioblastoma multiforme are not rare.
REF: Cancer 42:2854, 1978

786. Peripheral and cranial nerve damage caused by radiotherapy is not uncommon.
REF: Cancer 40:152, 1977

787. Neuroblastomas do not disseminate hematogenously.
REF: Ibid. , 39:2508

788. Postresection radiotherapy in patients with malignant
gliomas (astrocytoma grade IV) increases the survival
rate during the first year but does not influence the 5-
year survival.
REF: Ibid. , p. 873

789. In patients with incompletely resected astrocytomas
(grades I and II) and added postoperative irradiation, the
survival rate improved.
REF: Ibid.

790. Adriamycin (doxorubicin), an effective anticancer che-
motherapeutic agent, may selectively damage the dorsal
root ganglia resulting in ataxia.
REF: J. Neuropathol. Exp. Neurol. 36:907, 1977

791. Accumulation of neuromelanin within the cells of the substantia nigra reduces cytoplasmic RNA and gradually decreases the functional activity of the cell.
REF: Ibid. , p. 379

792. Meningiomas and nerve sheath tumors occur less frequently in Negroes than Caucasians.
REF: Ibid. , p. 41

793. Pituitary adenomas are more common in Negroes than in Caucasians.
REF: Ibid.

794. Glioblastoma multiforme is the most common individual primary CNS tumor.
REF: Ibid.

795. Gliomas are significantly more common in Caucasians than in Negroes.
REF: Ibid.

796. Primary CNS tumors are more common in American Negroes than in American Caucasians.
REF: Ibid.

797. Parkinsonism is often related to Von Economo's encephalitis, Japanese encephalitis and mild forms of chronic encephalitis of unknown etiology.
REF: Ibid. , 35:1

798. Periventricular leukomalacia is seen most commonly in the hypoxic premature.

799. Status marmoratus is a pathologic state primarily in the cerebral cortex of patients who have suffered traumatic insults in the first 2 years of life.

800. Ulegyria is an acquired lesion whereas polymicrogyria is a congenital lesion.

801. Congophilic angiopathy is a common cause of intracerebral hemorrhage in nonhypertensive aged patients.
REF: Arch. Pathol. Lab. Med. 102:317, 1978

802. An acute necrotizing hemorrhagic meningoencephalitis is typical of Naegleria Fowleri infection.
REF: Acta Neuropathol. 37:183, 1977

803. A muscle biopsy may be diagnostic in adult ceroid-lipo-fuscinosis (Kuf's disease).
REF: Acta Neuropathol. 45:67, 1979

804. Retrograde degeneration of the corticospinal tracts in man is a common finding at autopsy in compressive lesions of the spinal cord.
REF: Hum. Pathol. 9:602, 1978

805. Intracerebral metastases occur most frequently in the middle cerebral artery distribution and those from the most frequent primary sites usually are multiple.
REF: Burger, P. C. and Vogel, F. S.: Surgical Pathology of the Nervous System and Its Coverings, John Wiley and Sons, New York, 1976, p. 349

806. Astrocytomas are less common in the spinal cord than in the brain because spinal cord glia have a greater resistance to neoplastic transformation.
REF: Ibid., p. 512

807. Microtubules in nerves are involved in axonal sprouting and axoplasmic flow.
REF: Dyck, P. J., Thomas, P. K. and Lambert, E. H.: Peripheral Neuropathy, vol. I, W. B. Saunders Co., Philadelphia, 1975, p. 238

808. Most Schwann cells originate in the neural crest.
REF: Ibid., p. 201

809. Vasospasm-induced structural changes in cerebral arteries depend on the severity and duration of the vasospasm.
REF: Henderson, R. M., Boisvert, D. P. J. and Weir, B. K. A.: Adv. in Neurology, vol. 20, Raven Press, New York, 1978, p. 25

810. The cerebellar cortex shows dramatic changes in senescence.
REF: Res. Publ. Assoc. Res. in Nerv. Ment. Dis. 57:107, 1979

811. Persistence of the trigeminal artery is an uncommon developmental anomaly of little clinical significance.
REF: Lemire, R. J., et al.: Normal and Abnormal Development of the Nervous System, Harper & Row, Hagerstown, 1975, p. 329

ANSWERS AND COMMENTS

The author has made every effort to thoroughly verify the answers to the questions which appear on the preceding pages. However, as in any text, some inaccuracies and ambiguities may occur; therefore, if in doubt, please consult your references.

THE PUBLISHER

1. (D) The incidence is 12.1 per 100,000 in Rochester, Minnesota; it is more common in males, in older age groups, and with pre-existing hypertension.

2. (B) Sulcal enlargement and ventricular enlargement are common, infarcts and hemorrhages not infrequent, but subdurals did not occur in this series.

3. (C) Male brains weigh about 10% more than female brains on the average. Decline in brain weight begins near age 45.

4. (E) All are correct. Reduced absorption of calcium or changes in parathyroid function may not be necessary for development of bone disease in patients taking phenytoin.

5. (D) It is a persistent quivering, most often of the facial muscles, at times seen in polyradiculoneuropathy but more often with multiple sclerosis and brain stem tumors.

6. (E) Hemorrhage into the right thalamus was added to the other known sites causing unilateral neglect in a recent study; the dorsolateral frontal lobe is also a known site.

7. (D) It is usually symmetric (when bilateral), usually involves the globus pallidus, is usually not related to calcium disturbances and usually does not require further invasive studies.

8. (B) The number of selective injections is a marginally significant risk factor, and the presence of arterial stenosis greater than 90% is a strong risk factor.

9. (A) Higher "relative" work loads in normals caused a more pronounced elevation of lactate and creatine kinase. The other statements are true.

10. (C) In a large series, only 7 of 51 cases were diagnosed during life.

11. (B) They usually do not respond to ethosuximide (petit mal drug) and, at times, require temporal lobectomy for alleviation.

12. (C) Trimethadione is useful for petit mal, no help for grand mal. Phenytoin is not absorbed in intramuscular form.

13. (B) Autonomic neuropathy is also common; there is no known effective antidote.

14. (A) This has the earmarks of a progressive stroke which may proceed intermittently. We would favor the CT scan and LP and, if both showed no hemorrhage, treatment with IV heparin, but recently arteriography is being done more often with possible immediate carotid endartectomy and, it appears, with fewer catastrophic intracerebral hemorrhages than occurred 20 years ago when it was done in this situation.

15. (A) In this study of 195 patients, about 40% had electrophysiological alterations, showing a denervation pattern with generalized wasting.

16. (D) The trigeminal sensory root is second only to the sixth cranial nerve as a false localizing sign in cranial nerve involvement.

17. (C) Signs are often not impressive but are usually present in 50% of patients, and worsened with exercise in half of these.

18. (B) Half of the patients may be symptom-free after surgery, the rest will be improved. Surgical intervention is not urgent, however, as the disease progresses slowly.

19. (A) About 90% are simple, elementary, unilateral paresthetic seizures. They are frequently associated with focal motor seizures following the paresthesias and are always contralateral to the lesion.

20. (C) Occasionally the flexors of the forearm may be involved, usually the hand signs must be differentiated from lesions at the elbow or wrist.

21. (E) Most appear to be embolic; stump excision has been helpful at times.

22. (E) Occlusive extracranial disease occurred in less than 10%.

23. (A) The authors point out the problem should be further studied with the computerized tomography scan providing monitoring of efficacy.

24. (D) Probably the surgeon is the most important of these factors, operative mortality being less than 1% in several series.

25. (E) None of the three treatment regimens was superior to a group given only general supportive therapy in a randomized study.

26. (E) Cardiac arrhythmias and hyperlipidemia and possibly others should be added to this list.

27. (E) Benign epilepsy of childhood is not associated with encephalopathy and usually ends at puberty. Attacks may be rare or frequent, but are usually primary generalized in type.

28. (E) Magnesium sulfate is able to directly suppress neuronal burst firing and interictal spike generation at serum levels below those producing paralysis and thus interferes with this positive feedback system.

29. (D) The interval varied between 2 and 29 months. The authors believe this is consistent with a denervation supersensitivity hypothesis.

30. (A) Stomach-ache, nausea and vomiting may occur in 1/3 of patients, when the drug is given in the fasting state. These are usually transient and disappear after accommodation to the drug.

31. (B) In the older literature, the vermis was most commonly supposed damaged in speech disorders, but the superior portion of the left cerebellar hemisphere seems to be the area most commonly involved.

32. (C) A subacute onset, often with ascending paresthesias or leg weakness, offers the best prognosis while an acute onset, often with back pain, is worse. Preceding febrile illness, steroid treatment or CSF abnormalities, are not helpful prognostically.

33. (B) 37 out of 49 patients had VIII nerve involvement.

34. (A) The risk for children without prior neurologic disorder or atypical seizures is 2.5%, and is 17% for those with prior neurologic disorder.

35. (A) Unilateral frontal headaches were second most common.

36. (B) The mechanism of its action is unknown thus far.

37. (B) In 159 uses, it caused no death at this dosage, but did cause some hypotension.

38. (C) For some reason, diabetic nerves hold out better than normals when subjected to ischemia.

39. (D) It is said to increase transmitter release from motor nerve terminals by enhancing the influx of calcium ions through the nerve terminal membrane.

40. (E) They occur most often in older males, are dorsal and operation stops progression of the neurologic picture.

41. (C) There seems still to be some mystery surrounding this entity, both as to cause and pathology.

42. (A) Pure hemiparesis or hemiplegia was most consistent. Aphasia, when present, was transient.

43. (E) No statistically significant differences were noted in seizure control or acute side effects.

44. (E) Three pathologically verified cases illustrate this location.

45. (E) It increases excessively in some epileptics.

46. (D) Both are centrally represented, one or the other is also peripherally localized.

47. (C) Neither MS nor ALS patients had developed antibodies to a variety of arboviruses.

48. (A) The initial "peripheral" signs gave way to upper motor neuron long-term deficits.

49. (A) Memory disorders are early focal signs preceding more widespread intellectual deterioration.

50. (E) The lower rolandic area was more consistently involved than Broca's area with nonfluent aphasia.

51. (D) The prognosis was only slightly better for single metastasis cases.

52. (D) These disorders are all said to include defective central cholinergic function which is supplied by the two chemicals.

53. (C) High dose human leukocyte interferon limited cutaneous dissemination, visceral complications and progression within the primary dermatome.

54. (D) ACTH and anticonvulsants were both effective in a recent large series of cases. The EEG was most improved and in a dose-response relation.

55. (B) Major contributor to the middle trunk is C-7; C-5 and C-6 supply the upper trunk, and C-8 and T-1 supply the lower trunk.

56. (D) A similar, although transient change, occurs in hepatic encephalopathy contributing to an ever-enlarging role of neurotransmitters in disease.

57. (D) Demonstration of loss of cerebral blood flow is accepted as positive evidence of cerebral death. Only choice D reflects this occurrence.

58. (A) The peripheral neuropathy due to acute intermittent porphyria was found to be an axonal neuropathy on pathological study.

59. (B) This association has been noted in several recent studies and should lead to a cardiac work-up.

60. (D) EEG suppression bursts are generally associated with a poor prognosis while a lack of cerebral blood flow is proof of cerebral death. Clinical seizures have no relation to recovery.

61. (D) The psychosis also comes on years after the onset of seizures.

62. (E) There is no precise answer to this problem as yet.

63. (D) The differences in processing, as opposed to attention, are supported by the anatomic differences.

64. (B) If mild cases are included, the estimate rises to 11%.

65. (C) More people survive to the dementia-prone age range.

66. (B) A 2 per 1,000 prevalence has been proposed.

67. (A) Memory loss occurred in all, disorientation in 80%, agitation in 70%.

68. (C) Brain stem emboli were the most common complication in this series.

69. (E) All have been reported by several reviewers.

70. (E) Platelet aggregation to epinephrine decreases with the headache.

71. (B) There is abnormal skin pigmentation and probably abnormal fatty acid degradation.

72. (E) It may also have features of cerebellar degeneration.

73. (C) Dopamine hypersensitivity was noted only in patients with Shy-Drager syndrome.

74. (D) It remains unclear how blood pressure elevation produces headaches.

75. (B) As more persons live to an older age, a greater number of them seem to develop hypertensive encephalopathy, even though the overall incidence seems to be declining.

76. (A) The prevalence (2-3% in general autopsy series) has remained unchanged.

77. (E) Neurologic complications occur in under 5% with conventional doses, are mainly cerebellar in type, and relate to each individual dose more than to the total dose.

78. (A) Presumably, seeding of the epidural space or vertebral body occurs at the time of injury, possibly from an inapparent infection.

79. (D) These symptoms are associated with root involvement; spastic weakness with variable ataxia may result from cord involvement.

80. (A) Syringomyelia is irregularly progressive, making treatment modalities difficult to evaluate and is frequently associated with an aching, boring or lancinating pain, often severe in an analgesic limb.

81. (D) All of these peripheral neuropathies are primarily interstitial, rather than axonal, in type.

82. (D) This condition is associated with all the points mentioned.

83. (E) CPEO begins with ptosis, followed by symmetrical restriction of gaze in all directions. It may occur alone or in combination with a myriad of systemic or neurological signs.

84. (D) All three types of CSF can be seen following pituitary apoplexy. With repeated LP's, fluid initially normal tends later to fall into one of the other two groups.

85. (E) All may be present.

86. (C) The cause may be early uterine insult. It is not hereditary.

87. (D) She had Huntington's disease with lack of spontaneous speech, mild dementia, facial twitches and increased muscle tone characteristic of this disease in its young adult form.

88. (D) The ergot and barbiturate-analgesic mixture should both be stopped since they can be causing headaches if taken very regularly and daily.

89. (A) This is the usual onset.

90. (C) Dantrolene sodium was found effective in the treatment of malignant hyperpyrexia. Caffeine or calcium may cause worsening of the condition.

91. (E) Deanol helps erratically, if at all.

92. (C) It is more common in the northern tier of states. The etiology remains obscure, but it is probably acquired long before it becomes symptomatic, as suggested by migration studies.

93. (B) Papilledema and small ventricles are typical findings. Steroids help but medication for hypertension usually does not.

94. (B) Vasoconstrictors seem ineffective for this condition.

95. (C) This is not usually part of the constellation of signs and symptoms.

96. (E) All are treatable.

97. (C) Implants along the sciatic nerve may be the only involved area, although commonly it is more widespread.

98. (B) Bell's palsy is 3-4 times more common during pregnancy and 75% of the cases occur in the last trimester or immediately postpartum.

99. (C) Compression of the peroneal nerve at the knee by faulty positioning may produce identical symptoms.

100. (A) Headache and low neck pain without neurological signs are the most common presentation in most series, while isolated cranial nerve palsies (3, 5 and 7 most commonly) are in others.

101. (D) A very low glucose is characteristic, without which it is difficult to make the diagnosis, while the cell count and protein are more variable.

102. (B) Because a frontal lobe lesion may produce only personality disturbances and cerebellar lesions only obstruct CSF flow, they may not be detected until quite large.

103.   (A) The diagnosis should be suspect in any patient who is not severely obese and at menarche, menopause or with irregular menses, or who does not have a known cause.

104.   (D) Depending on the site of origin, jugular bulb, middle ear, or along the vagus nerve, these vascular tumors may cause multiple signs and symptoms.

105.   (C) Without treatment, 1/3 improve before delivery; 2/3 remit in the puerperium; 20% may have recurrences with later pregnancies.

106.   (D) This is according to the cooperative aneurysm study and does not apply to men. Cerebral venous thrombosis must be considered during pregnancy.

107.   (D) Two molecules of penicillamine combine with one atom of copper and are excreted in the urine. The introduction of this agent in 1956 was a great advance in treatment.

108.   (A) Its effectiveness may be restored with a drug "vacation".

109.   (E) The median and ulnar nerves are most likely entrapped.

110.   (F) Treatment appeared to help all types fairly evenly in this series.

111.   (C) Inappropriate rehydration of patients at risk appears to play a part.

112.   (A) Most well documented cases of ophthalmoplegic migraine have their onset from birth to age 11 years.

113.   (C) Most of the commonly used odor stimulants are effective in stimulating the trigeminal nerve, thus not as specific or useful in testing cranial nerve I.

114.   (A) Friedreich's ataxia is autosomal recessive in the majority of cases.

115.   (C) Several recent studies show that sensory evoked potentials are abnormal in the majority of patients. Significantly, this includes a large number of patients who do not have clinical deficits related to the system under test.

116. (C) For unknown reasons, adenocarcinomas of the lung and stomach are consistently reported as the most common tumor forms.

117. (C) The incidence is 17 times greater than expected when both are present.

118. (D) Two cases are described with right hemisphere dominance for affective speech.

119. (C) Though unusual, they do occur in both forms.

120. (B) Patients with severe "on-off" phenomena could not tolerate bromocriptine. Benefit from 70 mgs. daily of bromocriptine was comparable to 750 mgs. of L-dopa with carbidopa.

121. (C) A large series review provided these figures.

122. (A) Hypothalamic symptoms were surprisingly infrequent; increased intracranial pressure and Parinaud's syndrome were common.

123. (B) The opiate antagonist, naltrexane, had no effect, but the analogs of aporphines along with Sinemet[R] improved some refractory patients.

124. (D) "Release" hallucinations begin after a postinsult latent period, and tend to be more continuous than epileptic visual phenomena.

125. (B) The degree of functional impairment, and not evident structural change per se, seems to be the more important factor in survival.

126. (C) Hesitant, stuttering dysarthric and dysphasic speech is the most characteristic feature of this disease, and is often combined with dementia, myoclonus and seizures. The EEG is usually more abnormal than would be expected clinically.

127. (C) Recent clinical/anatomical studies have shown the syndrome may be caused by unilateral, nondominant posterior hemispheric lesions, as well as the more usually reported bilateral posterior-inferior occipitotemporal lesions.

128. (C) A study of 49 patients suggests both factors are important.

129. (D) Neither the occurrence of nystagmus nor the degree of lateral gaze at onset correlates reliably with phenytoin blood levels.

130. (C) The alcohol excess factor was found in a Finnish study of unexpected strokes in young people.

131. (C) Phenothiazines help the psychiatric symptoms. Glucose may help to suppress induction of ALA synthetase.

132. (C) Several studies confirm these findings.

133. (B) The CSF globulins are not usually elevated.

134. (B) It identifies organisms and certain subtypes but provides no direct evidence for drug sensitivity.

135. (A) Herpes simplex virus is the only agent causing encephalitis consistently responsive to vidarabine.

136. (C) Both types are recognized, among others.

137. (A) Flucytosine is useful as adjunct therapy; amphotericin B is the most effective agent.

138. (D) Detection of seizure discharge on the EEG to confirm the clinical suspicion is a sampling problem, since seizure activity on the EEG occurs at unpredictable times. A repeat tracing should be obtained if treatment decisions cannot be made on clinical grounds.

139. (C) A sixth nerve palsy is a well known false localizing sign which is rarely present, but the inferonasal field cut, though even more rare, may result from nonspecific increased intracranial pressure. It must be remembered that, most commonly, neither sign is present.

140. (C) Low serum magnesium levels may be associated with neuromuscular hyperexcitability (seizures, tremor, etc.) and other behavioral disturbances, (irritability, depression, etc.).

141.   (A) About 75% improve, while the rest stay the same or worsen. Ergotamines have an oxytocic effect on the uterus and should be avoided (ergotamine tartrate given orally supposedly does not, but probably should be avoided).

142.   (B) About 10% of myasthenics have associated hyperthyroidism, though the converse is much rarer.

143.   (B) Usually associated with low serum potassium.

144.   (A) Ataxia may be the presenting symptom, with truncal difficulties usually worse than appendicular problems.

145.   (C) About 40% of women worsen just before menses; this improves in about half after thymectomy.

146.   (C) Nalidixic acid is the most common antibiotic associated with this syndrome; vitamin A was first discovered as a cause in Arctic explorers eating polar bear liver.

147.   (F) No. They are fair screening tests but will miss significant lesions.

148.   (F) No relationship has been found.

149.   (F) It is usually normal; pathologic changes are usually distal and nerve roots are spared.

150.   (F) It may produce temporary improvement.

151.   (T) There are usually other signs and symptoms of drug toxicity as well.

152.   (T) A placebo double blind study has possibly laid the serpents to rest.

153.   (F) A combination of the substrate for glutamic acid dehydrogenase and its cofactor did nothing to stop this disease of GABA deficiency.

154.   (T) Newer therapy with vidarabine apparently changes this dismal outlook.

155.   (F) It improved the functional status of the patients also.

156.   (F) Transient stuttering is associated with unilateral (left) lesions, permanent with bilateral.

157. (T) The IgM is apparently not related to measles anti-bodies.

158. (T) It did produce other signs of probably central cholin-ergic stimulation, however.

159. (T) The prognosis for life has also improved considerably in the last few decades.

160. (F) They are rapid in onset, the maximum being attained usually in less than a minute.

161. (T) Longer episodes, up to 24 hours, are distinctly less common.

162. (T) Cost is reduced considerably, however, if the acute care is in the community hospital with referral later on to the rehabilitation center.

163. (F) It improved survival in this study.

164. (T) Alzheimer's disease is several times more common than stroke in causing dementia.

165. (T) It is not a proven relationship.

166. (F) In this study, they were nearly identical in all im-portant respects.

167. (F) The authors believe it is secondary to operative trau-ma to the carotid vessel or sheath.

168. (F) Improved control of hypertension is probably responsible.

169. (F) Several centers are having good success operating on an emergency basis after arteriography without, so far, the heretofore expected complications.

170. (T) This is due to the excessive distance that the regen-erating axons must travel, thus resulting in severe at-rophy of the intrinsic hand muscles.

171. (F) Present surgical techniques cannot adequately re-pair severed roots with traumatic meningoceles.

172. (T) These lesions usually affect young men who have good rehabilitation potential.

173. (F) Primary cerebral amyloid angiopathy is an important cause of mental deterioration and fatal cerebral hemorrhages in the elderly, but bears no direct relationship to the severity of either cerebral or visceral atherosclerosis.

174. (F) Such a study is needed, even though a small series of patients managed medically for one month to 6 years had rather benign courses.

175. (T) The trigeminal nerve innervates the basal meninges of the anterior and middle fossae, and the reactivated virus may spread along the fifth nerve fibers.

176. (F) It is fairly common, 15% of cases being familial in a worldwide survey.

177. (F) Occipital lobe AVM's usually produce strictly unilateral headaches (migraine switches sides with repeated attacks) and brief, episodic, unformed visual phenomena without the angular, scintillating figures experienced with migraine.

178. (T) Medical treatment of blepharospasm with anticholinergics, haldol, and others frequently fails and one has to resort to differential facial nerve section if the case is severe. Clonazepam has recently been used successfully in a few cases, with larger trials needed to establish overall efficacy.

179. (F) Both may slow the evoked responses.

180. (F) No decrement in IQ or early academic performance was found.

181. (T) There is a possibility that both disorders may have presymptomatic carriers of "slow virus".

182. (T) In this case report, the encephalomyelitis was retreated with adenine arabinoside and then with prednisone with some response.

183. (T) Most infants and children with true febrile convulsions have other family members with similar generalized convulsions precipitated by fever at varying elevations.

184. (F) In an English study, recurrent optic neuritis was as significant as demyelination elsewhere in predicting M. S.

185.   (T) The patient has little disturbance of awareness, but has interrupted corticobulbar and corticospinal pathways.

186.   (F) The long half-life of phenobarbital makes once or twice daily therapy possible.

187.   (T) Children do not usually remember these in the morning, and tend to outgrow them.

188.   (T) Both NREM and REM sleep are decreased.

189.   (F) Seizures are rare sequelae of thrombotic strokes, but occur in more than 20 percent of embolic episodes.

190.   (F) On the contrary, theoretically they may shunt blood away from diseased low flow areas.

191.   (F) The margin is, in fact, very narrow and accounts for an occasional fatality in alcoholic intoxication.

192.   (T) Also called the uremic twitch convulsive syndrome, this is usually associated with renal failure even though the primary disease may be systemic.

193.   (T) It is usually lost only if the patient has suffered hypoxic damage.

194.   (F) Originally, this was thought to be so, but most neurologists now agree it is a rare or late mode of presentation.

195.   (T) According to McAlpine's study, a further 20% relapse in 5-9 years and another 10% in 10-30 years.

196.   (F) This entity is in doubt, but the form of parkinsonism subsequent to strokes is characterized by corticospinal tract signs, increased reflexes, and spastic bulbar palsy.

197.   (F) The onset is most commonly in the sixth decade with loss of voluntary eye movements, loss of Bell's phenomenon, pseudobulbary palsy and axial dystonia.

198.   (T) The explanation for this clinical and pathological sparing is entirely unknown.

199.   (T) The rate varies from 0.5 to 1.4 from country to country except for the foci in Guam, New Guinea and Japan where it is much higher.

200. (T) Downward gaze weakness is followed by weakness of upward gaze and then total ophthalmoplegia.

201. (T) Usually this cataract is posterior subcapsular.

202. (F) It commonly causes a mild transient leukopenia.

203. (F) It occurs mainly in males, but the bulbar type is the most severe.

204. (F) Moderate doses (80-160 mg/day) seem to be more effective.

205. (F) This is probably compression of the peroneal nerve by leg crossing in a person who has recently lost weight and now, with thinner thighs, can traumatize the nerve between the fibula and patella.

206. (T) This is common and the patient can be reassured.

207. (T) True, especially in young adults and children.

208. (T) This type of stroke may not manifest completely and any of these may be the presenting complaint to the neurologist. Look for the Horner's syndrome in a dim light.

209. (F) The potential for addiction to alcohol is increased because it works so well.

210. (T) Chronic inhalation may produce a mysterious neurologic picture which may be related to vitamin B_{12} deficiency syndromes.

211. (T) That is usually the case. Most patients interpret field defects as loss of vision in one eye.

212. (T) If there is no EOM or lid weakness, it will probably turn out to be some other disease.

213. (F) Rapid ALS can raise the enzymes somewhat.

214. (T) Many physicians use this approach.

215. (F) Most patients find out quickly that alcohol will trigger the headache.

216. (F) It may stay between 3000 to 4000 with this drug and not go lower. It is worrisome, however, and should be watched.

217. (T) True, particularly after an apparently insignificant injury.

218. (T) It has been so reported and also after nothing at all.

219. (F) In our opinion, it is a fairly reliable sign.

220. (T) As an isolated complaint, it means nothing.

221. (F) The episodes are too short. Look for causes of compression of the ulnar nerve.

222. (T) CNS fatigue with use is common, in fact the expected thing, with M. S.

223. (T) Multiple causes of "ulnar neuropathy" appear to be more common than single ones.

224. (F) It probably plays a part. This is one of the big problems with the current use of these medications in the long term treatment of parkinsonism. They may have to be stopped completely.

225. B
226. D
227. C
228. A
229. C
230. B
231. A
232. B
233. A
234. C
235. (C) Both produce combined ulnar and median nerve palsy with loss of sensation in the medial aspect of the hand, forearm and arm.

236. (A) Infant botulism is characterized clinically by extreme weakness and inability to suck or swallow. Pupillary and deep tendon reflexes may be retained.

237. (E) Fisher's syndrome is a benign disease with complete recovery. It is manifest clinically by ataxia, external ophthalmoplegia and areflexia. The etiology is unknown.

238. (A) This syndrome consists of a triad of recurrent facial paralyses, edema of face and lips and a furrowed tongue.

239. (E) Depressed serum ceruloplasmin levels and increased urinary copper excretion are found in other causes of chronic liver disease. A liver biopsy for determination of hepatic copper content is necessary for the diagnosis of Wilson's disease.

240. (D) Infants under 6 months of age with Reye's syndrome are usually from the lower socioeconomic urban areas. Sudden onset of respiratory distress with apnea is a characteristic finding.

241. (C) The smooth, small tongue with absent fungiform papillae is present in the neonate. Excessive sweating does not become evident until after one month of age.

242. (E) Drug ingestion always has to be considered in a child with an unexplained altered state of consciousness.

243. (E) Abnormal development or neurologic status and complex febrile seizures greatly enhance the probability of developing a seizure disorder.

244. (D) Gelastic seizures may be associated with lesions (tumors) of the temporal lobe, limbic system or posterior hypothalamus. They are rare in children.

245. (E) I-cell disease is thought to be a result of a deficit of neuraminidase.

246. (E) The true incidence of seizure headaches is unknown, but probably is greater than recognized at present.

247. (A) Various studies quote such a range of incidences in children coming to medical centers as a result of head trauma. Obviously, the definition of "significant head injury" affects these figures.

248. (C) The effectiveness of DPH therapy in migraine has
      been shown in a number of recent studies. The basis for
      this is obscure. The lack of correlation with EEG sei-
      zure discharges as shown in a recent study suggests that
      it may not be related to the anticonvulsant effect.

249. (E) The younger the child at the time of the insult result-
      ing in aphasia, the more likely is the child to have com-
      plete recovery.

250. (D) All imply a serious prognosis.

251. (B) Hunter's syndrome is transmitted as a sex-linked
      recessive.

252. (D) Scheie's syndrome is compatible with survival into
      late adulthood and normal intelligence.

253. (B) The onset of massive spasm is usually between 1-13
      months, and most often before 6 months of age.

254. (E) Most cases thus far described have been in Cauca-
      sians, many of Scandinavian origin.

255. (E) The listed reflexes are brain stem reflexes and can
      be elicited in infants with absent cerebral hemispheres
      (anencephalic monster). The one neonatal reflex that re-
      quires cortical function is fixing and following.

256. (E) Usually, the migrainous attack begins with severe
      onset of a throbbing headache. Scotomas may be noted
      in children over 10 years of age. 50% of all migraine
      begins before 16 years of age.

257. (E) It is a prominent feature of all the listed conditions.

258. (D) Narcolepsy is uncommon in early childhood but fre-
      quently appears during the teenage years. 5% of patients
      have difficulty before age 10.

259. (E) The cherry red spot is the result of degeneration of
      ganglion cells surrounding the fovea. The vascular sup-
      ply of the choroid is then observed as a reddened area
      encircled by a gray ring.

260. (A) Preferential handedness before 18 months of age
      raises the suspicion of opposite hand and arm weakness
      or spasticity.

261. (C) The Landau reflex is not present until age 10 months.

262. (E) The diseases secondary to abnormal amino acid metabolism characteristically produce seizures in the newborn period.

263. (D) Tyrosine levels are low normal in phenylketonuria. The tyrosine levels are much higher than the phenylalanine levels in phenylalaninemia of premature and immature infants.

264. (A) This is an autosomal recessive disease due to a defect in branched-chain amino acid metabolism and occurs in both Caucasian and black patients. Structural alterations are limited to cerebral white matter.

265. (E) Children with myasthenia gravis respond less well to medicine than adults but are less likely to have respiratory distress.

266. (C) Seizures are the most common manifestation of pyridoxine deficiency in infancy.

267. (C) A normal infant will usually transfer objects by 28 weeks.

268. (D) Hypocalcemia in the first 24-48 hours of life has been associated with hypoxia, prematurity, maternal parathyroid disease and causes not yet delineated.

269. (E) Holoprosencephaly is characterized by small head, hypotelorism and midline facial defects.

270. (C) The diagnosis of neurofibromatosis can be made at any age if six or more cafe-au-lait spots measuring 1.5 cm. in diameter are present.

271. (C) Herpes most often involves the temporal lobe.

272. (A) Hydrocephalus is a common finding in patients with myelomeningocele. If the myelomeningocele is in the thoracolumbar area, 97% of the patients will have hydrocephalus.

273. (D) A circumference below 32 cm. is small and a circumference of 30 cm. or below is grossly abnormal.

274. (D) Krabbe's (globoid leukodystrophy) is associated with a small head.

275. (E) Congenital malformations of the central nervous system are not usually associated with seizures in the first six weeks of life.

276. (E) The primary pathology in Guillain-Barre syndrome is in the anterior roots.

277. (D) 80% of patients are deficient in IgE. There is a high incidence of pulmonary infection in patients with ataxia telangiectasia.

278. (D) The history of intolerance to milk and jaundice coupled with the physical findings of hepatomegaly, cataracts and developmental retardation is classical for galactosemia.

279. (E) Galactosemia is diagnosed by the absence of galactose-1-phosphate uridyl transferase.

280. (B) A rate of growth that exceeds 1.5 cm./month is abnormal.

281. (C) Metachromatic leukodystrophy is associated with both central white matter and peripheral nerve involvement.

282. (A) The spinal fluid protein is usually normal in SSPE. The CSF gamma globulin is elevated.

283. (C) The ash leaf lesion is present at birth. Adenoma sebaceum does not occur until after 18 months of age. Subungual fibromas do not appear until puberty.

284. (C) A young child with stumbling gait, increasing ataxia and associated slurred speech should be considered to have a posterior fossa tumor.

285. (C) Massive spasm may be associated with several disease entities but most commonly results from neonatal hypoxia.

286. (E) Sydenham's chorea is characterized by emotional lability, muscle weakness and purposeless movements. The child is unable to stick his tongue out and keep it out (Jack-in-box tongue).

287. (E) The only findings common in all patients with reflex sympathetic dystrophy are dysesthesia and hyperesthesia. Other symptoms include edema, cyanosis and hyperhidrosis.

288. (E) Failure of adequate brain growth after birth has been associated with hypoxia, hypoglycemia, polycythemia and central nervous system infection. Hypoxia is probably the most common cause of an acquired small head.

289. B
290. D
291. A
292. C
293. D
294. F
295. G
296. B
297. D
298. C
299. I
300. H
301. A
302. E
303. B
304. D
305. C
306. A
307. E

308. (T) Fibromuscular dysplasia has recently been reported as a cause of stroke in infancy and childhood.

309. (T) 21/15 translocation occurs more commonly in the young mother and accounts for the increased likelihood of a second mongoloid child in women under 25.

310. (F) Patients treated with copper have shown no improvement.

311. (T) Early diagnosis of homocystinuria is important as most patients respond to pyridoxine or pyridoxine and folic acid.

312. (T) The reduction in lung volume correlates only with intrauterine onset of disease and not to the degree of muscle weakness or the duration of the disease.

313. (T) Most intracranial AV malformations are associated with an intracranial bruit in the young infant.

314. (F) Intracranial bruits are common in children over 4 months of age and under 3 years of age.

315. (T) Tuberous sclerosis, Aicardi syndrome and gyral malformations are common in infants with infantile spasms.

316. (F) The sooner after birth the epilepsy begins the worse the prognosis.

317. (T) It is probably not needed.

318. (T) Recent reports confirm this.

319. (T) Vincristine and methotrexate do potentiate the neurotoxic effects of CNS irradiation. This is of major clinical concern since combined chemotherapy and irradiation to the central nervous system are being used with increasing frequency.

320. (T) The disorder apparently improves with or without treatment.

321. (T) The differential diagnosis of anosmia is diverse. Unilateral anosmia is of greater concern than bilateral anosmia.

322. (T) Fifty percent of children who have febrile seizures have only one seizure. Usually, prophylactic treatment is not begun until the child has a second febrile seizure.

323. (T) The child with Down's syndrome has a normal head circumference at birth.

324. (F) Less than 5% of patients with tuberous sclerosis have rhabdomyomas of the heart, but 50% of patients who have rhabdomyomas of the heart have tuberous sclerosis.

325. (T) Only 2/3 of all children manifesting symptoms of hyperactivity respond to stimulant therapy.

326. (F) Wilson's disease in the pediatric patient usually presents as a chronic active hepatitis. Kayser-Fleischer rings may be absent.

327.   (T) If the child presents with neurologic signs, Kayser-Fleischer rings will be present. Diagnosis may be made by slit-lamp examination.

328.   (T) The majority of children with Wilson's disease respond to treatment with D-Penicillamine.

329.   (T) Seizures commonly present as vertigo. A majority of these children have unilateral or bilateral paroxysmal temporal lobe discharges on EEG.

330.   (T) The absence of cytochrome C oxidase activity in peripheral muscle tissue causes the increase of the mitochondrial NADH/NAD ratio as reflected by the frequently elevated beta-hydroxybutyrate/acetoacetate ratio in the blood.

331.   (F) Sodium benzoate lowers the blood glycine level and decreases the CSF glycine level but does not lower the CSF glycine level to normal.

332.   (T) The clinical course of acetaminophen poisoning is so similar to Reye's syndrome that it is conceivable that many children considered to have Reye's syndrome actually have acetaminophen poisoning.

333.   (T) Abnormal valine metabolism has rarely been implicated in the development of neurologic symptoms. Leucine is the major cause of the neurologic symptoms associated with maple syrup urine disease. A new variant has been described in which valine is responsible for the neurologic symptoms.

334.   (T) In the hyperphenylalaninemic variants, slightly elevated phenylalanine levels exist early in life but do not require treatment with a low phenylalanine diet.

335.   (F) The risk of SSPE following vaccination appears less than the risk following natural measles.

336.   (F) SSPE is a complication of early measles. 46% have a history of measles before the second birthday.

337.   (T) 19% of patients with factor VII deficiency have intracranial bleeding.

338.   (F) Transcutaneous nerve stimulation in many instances completely relieves the pain of reflex sympathetic dystrophy. This may be the preferred treatment for this condition.

339.   (T) PAS stained smears reveal large glycogen granules in the lymphocytes. PAS positive granules are not specific for any disease but are supportive evidence for the diagnosis of Pompe's disease.

340.   (F) Several large studies indicate that the incidence of subsequent afebrile seizures is approximately 2 to 3%, which is a sixfold increase compared to the general population.

341.   (T) The majority of recurrent febrile seizures will occur within 30 months of the onset of the disorder. Therefore, therapy can probably be discontinued after 30 months.

342.   (T) The administration of glycine prevents the expected rise of blood isovaleric acid following oral leucine load. Glycine and isovaleric acid react in liver and kidney to form a nontoxic conjugate, isovalerylglycine, which is rapidly excreted into the urine.

343.   (T) Seizures may develop immediately after head injury or after an interval of months to years. If seizures occur early (within 4 days after injury) there is an 8% incidence of recurrent late seizures.

344.   (T) They do occur in 0.5% of all children, but 2-3% of all children have febrile seizures.

345.   (T) The primary defect in citrullinemia is a deficiency or absence of this enzyme. Urea synthesis is impaired but the blood urea levels are normal.

346.   (F) Seizures are not common and usually are controlled by decrease in phenylalanine intake.

347.   (T) Pelizaeus-Merzbacher is a rare leukodystrophy with early onset in infancy. The prominent clinical feature does consist of pendular oscillation of the globes in combination with titubation of the head.

348.   (F) Akinetic seizures are associated with loss of postural tone.

349. (B) This often recurrent neuropathy characteristically elevates the CSF protein and responds dramatically to steroids.

350. (A) The percentage of malignancy associated with polymyositis is 10-17%, somewhat lower than once thought.

351. (B) Raynaud's phenomenon is seen in approximately 1/3 of patients.

352. (A) The prevalence rate of myasthenia gravis is one in 10, 000 to one in 50, 000; it begins later in males as a rule.

353. (A) Usually, in inherited sensory neuropathy type I, the primary abnormalities are in unmyelinated fibers.

354. (D) Diabetic peripheral neuropathy is produced by multiple factors.

355. (D) All conditions mentioned give rise to axonal forms of neuropathy.

356. (A) Neonatal transient myasthenia gravis occurs in infants born to mothers who have the disease. The symptoms may last for 1 month. It is not related to the duration of the disease in the mother nor to the type of treatment in the mother.

357. (E) Neonatal persistent myasthenia gravis occurs in infants born to mothers who do not have the disease. The symptoms are milder than in the juvenile form and respiratory dysfunction is not common. There is relative resistance to drug therapy.

358. (D) Prognosis in the congenital form usually tends to be good. Greater incapacity is observed in the late onset form.

359. (E) Triglyceride levels increase after a prolonged fast. Usually, these patients, after fasting for 10 to 12 hours, have markedly increased ketone bodies in the urine and marked ketonuria develops after oral meals containing medium chain triglycerides.

360. (A) Talwin may produce muscle stiffness due to fibrosis.

361. (D) Paramyotonia congenita is often associated with paradoxical response to exercise. When a patient exercises, instead of the muscles getting looser or stronger they get weak, contrary to other forms of myotonia.

362. (D) There are three types of onset of facio-scapulo-humeral muscular dystrophy.

363. (D) All three characterize this entity.

364. (A) Patients respond well to phenytoin and not very well to quinine and procainamide. The reasons for this response are poorly understood.

365. (A) Diabetes is associated with marked autonomic dysfunction, the others less so.

366. (D) Muscle histology and histochemistry are most diagnostic; abnormalities in the other tests are seen in other conditions as well.

367. (C) The other treatments mentioned do not improve the conduction velocities as much.

368. (B) Of these muscle storage disorders, McArdle's disease is characterized by marked myoglobinuria, the others less so.

369. (C) These patients have myoglobinuria following exercise and do not have any muscle atrophy or fasciculations.

370. (A) They are not usually seen in chronic neuropathy or facio-scapulo-humeral muscular dystrophy.

371. (C) Cardiac tissue is involved most severely and consistently in myotonic dystrophy.

372. (A) The abnormalities in acetylcholine receptor protein at postsynaptic levels have been very well delineated.

373. (C) It is not a muscle disease as was thought in the past.

374. (C) Distal muscle weakness is characteristic of myotonic dystrophy. Proximal muscle weakness is characteristic of the other dystrophies listed.

375. (D) Pseudohypertrophy has been reported in all the muscular dystrophies except myotonic dystrophy. Pseudohypertrophy also occurs with polymyositis.

376. (A) This type of neuropathy is inherited in a dominant fashion.

377. (A) Duchenne muscular dystrophy is the most common type.

378. (B) This form of spinal muscular atrophy is inherited predominantly as an autosomal dominant trait.

379. (A) Lupus is the most likely cause although mononeuritis multiplex may occur with all of the listed conditions.

380. (A) Central fascicular demyelination of the oculomotor nerve spares the outer region where the pupillomotor fibers are located.

381. (C) The other conditions are prevalent in certain areas but leprosy is still the most common world-wide.

382. (A) Hereditary amyloid neuropathy is transmitted in autosomal dominant fashion.

383. (A) Myotonia in this disorder can be eliminated after the nerve is blocked by curarization.

384. (C) Both are correct.

385. (C) There are two types of myotonia congenita; Thompson's form of myotonia congenita is autosomal dominant, but Becker's type is recessive.

386. (T) Malignant hyperpyrexia has recently been reported in association with Schwartz-Jampel syndrome.

387. (F) This usually subclinical nerve dysfunction is probably another manifestation of this multisystem disease, independent of glucose intolerance.

388. (T) Females are more prone to have polymyositis than males.

389. (F) The lower extremity muscles are affected earlier than the upper extremity muscles.

390. (T) Abnormalities in various immunoglobulins are noted in 50% of cases with polymyositis.

391. (T) There are various abnormalities postulated in the etiology of polymyositis; one is delayed hypersensitivity.

392. (F) Percentagewise, polymyalgia rheumatica is seen more in elderly females than in males.

393. (T) Conventional medical treatment is not very effective with coexistent thymoma.

394. (F) Usually, the extensor muscles are more affected than the flexor muscles in myasthenia gravis.

395. (T) 7-10% of mothers with myasthenia have myasthenic infants.

396. (F) 99% of cases with this disorder occur in adult life, between the third and seventh decades.

397. (T) Rarely, sensory nerve conduction may not show any abnormalities, but there is a prolonged distal motor latency; usually, however, there is sensory slowing with or prior to motor slowing.

398. (T) It is an autosomal dominant disease.

399. (T) Neurophysiological data support this fact.

400. (T) Older patients have prolonged EMG motor unit potentials.

401. (F) Fibrillation potentials are not only seen in denervated muscles, but are also seen in dystrophies, polymyositis, etc.

402. (T) Patients with myopathic conditions have these abnormal potentials, but they are not diagnostic of any single disorder.

403. (C) They were found in 87% of unselected patients and usually are unrelated to blood pressure.

404. (A) They may be abnormal in other conditions, even in patients without a history of optic neuritis.

405.   (C) It was far more common in drug-induced coma than in the other conditions.

406.   (E) It may be present with neocortical death despite absent visual evoked responses.

407.   (E) Skew deviation has been reported secondary to lesions in all three divisions of the brain stem, being statistically more frequent with lesions in the pons (61%).

408.   (D) Extraocular muscle palsies have been reported to occur in from 7% to 31% of cases of herpes zoster ophthalmicus. In decreasing order of frequency, this is secondary to dysfunction of the third, sixth, and fourth cranial nerves.

409.   (D) Drusen are refractile, granular bodies buried within the optic disc. They tend to occur in congenitally "full" dysplastic discs, which have the erroneous appearance of papilledema. Retinal hemorrhage may occur; 71% of affected eyes develop field defects.

410.   (C) Strictly ocular symptoms without bulbar or skeletal involvement constitute group I of adult myasthenia and represent 20% of all patients with M. G.

411.   (C) Duane's syndrome is a congenital syndrome of anomalous ocular muscle cofiring.

412.   (B) 2/3 of parkinsonian patients may show prolonged VEP's, depending on the type of stimulation parameters. Some patients' VEP latency improves after levodopa therapy.

413.   (A) Although rarer than optic nerve damage, ophthalmoplegia occurs in about 10% of cases, usually before visual impairment. Pathologically, extraocular muscle infarcts are seen.

414.   (D) There is a generalized structural and functional abnormality of mitochondria involving ocular and somatic muscle, sweat glands, liver cells, peripheral and central neural tissue, and undoubtedly other organs as well.

415.   (D) Other causes include the Sylvian aqueduct syndrome, bilateral blindness from retinal or optic nerve lesions, alcoholism with Wernicke's encephalopathy, multiple sclerosis, etc.

416. (E) Oculosympathetic fibers innervate the muscles of Muller in the upper and lower lids, resulting in drooping of the upper lid (ptosis) and elevation of the lower lid ("upside down" ptosis), with apparent enophthalmos, when the fibers are not functioning.

417. (B) Along with acute evanescent disc swelling, this is characteristic of ischemic optic neuropathy. An ESR should differentiate the idiopathic from the arteritic variety.

418. (D) It also may occur in progressive supranuclear palsy, Wilson's disease, mesodiencephalic junction neoplasms, Whipple's disease, progressive multifocal leukoencephalopathy, and ataxia telangiectasia.

419. (A) Opsoclonus occurs in association with a number of conditions. It is often continuous and does occur when the eyes are closed. It is often seen as a distant neurologic effect of a neuroblastoma.

420. (C) Fibers which subserve the so-called "temporal crescent" (fibers carrying information from the extreme temporal field, $60-90^\circ$) can be traced to their destination in the opposite, most anterior mesial occipital lobe. Lesions of the posterior occipital lobe may spare this "temporal crescent".

421. (D) Many toxins have given rise to bilateral cecocentral scotomas from bilateral toxic optic neuropathy. For a more complete list, consult the reference.

422. (D) Organic causes of bilateral concentric narrowing of the fields include end stage retinitis pigmentosa and glaucoma, bilateral occipital lobe infarcts with bimacular sparing, and postpapilledema optic atrophy.

423. (A) It is the only type of nystagmus which is specifically related to cerebellar dysfunction.

424. (B) It is a relatively specific sign of severe pontine involvement (hemorrhage or infarction, either primary or from extrinsic pressure).

425. (A) Simultaneous quantitative recordings of head and eye movements in a patient with spasmus nutans showed the head movements to be compensatory, tending to abolish the abnormal ocular oscillation.

426. (C) There is a blockage in orthograde and retrograde axonal transport at the optic disc. This leads to an accumulation of axonal content, axonal swelling, and the eventual increase in disc volume clinically recognized as papilledema.

427. (C) Optic nerve lesions of diverse etiologies tend to affect preferentially the central core of axons in the nerve, the papillomacular bundle. Central or cecocentral scotomas are then the most usual field defect.

428. (A) In one-fourth of the cases, the optic nerve involvement and myelitis occur simultaneously, and in one-fourth the optic nerve involvement precedes the myelitis.

429. (C) The flocculus receives both primary afferent vestibular input and, at least in lower animals, visual feedback via the accessory optic tract. Efferent floccular outflow then appropriately adjusts excitation/inhibition of vestibulo-ocular relay neurons.

430. (B) See-saw nystagmus refers to this pattern, with repetition of this sequence in the opposite direction providing the see-saw effect. Upper brain stem pathology due to compression from large chiasmal tumors or due to vascular disease has been noted.

431. B
432. A
433. C

434. (C) Both unilateral and bilateral lesions have been reported to cause paralysis of downgaze.

435. (B) Voluntary horizontal gaze is defective; agenesis of the corpus callosum is found in some patients.

436. (B) Apparently, the CNS can control the firing frequencies and recruitment of motoneurons more precisely than it can control the duration of the high-frequency motoneuronal saccadic burst.

437. (C) Neonatal myasthenia is a well known cause. Fluctuating ophthalmoplegia has also been reported with various newborn metabolic abnormalities such as branched-chain aminoaciduria and nonketotic hyperglycinemia.

438. (C) Lower lid retraction is seen with Graves' disease, central or peripheral facial paresis, myasthenia, myopathies, proptosis, and ectropion.

439. (A) Ocular signs which may occur secondary to clostridium botulinum infection include bilateral ptosis, progressive ophthalmoplegia, and dilated, poorly reactive pupils.

440. (C) Intracavernous lesions may give rise to parasympathetic or sympathetic pupillary involvement, in which case, anisocoria is the rule. Not infrequently, however, sympathetic and parasympathetic deficits coexist in these patients, and isocoria may result with uniform background illumination.

441. (B) Pattern VER using varying size checkerboard patterns can be used to estimate infant acuity, but flash VER cannot. OKN response to progressively smaller stripe patterns is useful in estimating infant acuity.

442. (B) The cerebellum has been found paramount in the generation of smooth pursuit eye movements. Defective or "cogwheel" pursuit has been a consistent finding, with floccular lesions appearing to be the specific area responsible for these deficits.

443. (A) This rare syndrome is frequently noted at birth or within the first year of life, and is associated with congenital or infantile oculomotor nerve palsies.

444. (A) Latent nystagmus is a jerk form of nystagmus present only when one eye is covered, with the fast phase toward the uncovered eye. It is always congenital.

445. (B) The regeneration of visual pigment after bleaching with a bright light stimulus is unimpaired in patients with optic nerve disease, but is usually deficient in patients with macular pathology.

446. (C) Deep excavations of the optic disc resulting from incomplete closure of the fetal optic fissure may be associated with congenital malformations of other midline structures, including basal encephalocele with or without pulsating exophthalmos.

447. (C) They present with progressive visual loss and axial proptosis. Initial unilateral mild disc edema is often seen, followed by optic atrophy.

448. (B) Bi-horizontal jerk nystagmus secondary to drug abuse is frequently seen. With increasing toxicity, gaze evoked upbeat nystagmus is also seen, but gaze evoked nystagmus in downgaze is rare.

449. (C) Incongruous homonymous field defects usually indicate optic tract lesions. Although rare, lateral geniculate lesions can also give rise to such field defects.

450. (A) Horizontal jerk nystagmus for approximately 90 seconds followed by a 10 second neutral phase, with 90 seconds of horizontal jerk nystagmus in the opposite direction forms the basic pattern. Lesions of the lower brain stem are usually responsible.

451. (C) Bilateral occipital dysfunction is the usual substrate underlying cortical blindness. Hypoxia, ictal inhibitory seizures and postictal phenomena are included among the many potential etiologies.

452. (A) Lid retraction and lid lag (not ptosis), proptosis, and extraocular muscle restrictions are the most frequent eye signs in Graves' disease. Stare with infrequent blinking may also occur. For a complete list, consult reference.

453. (A) The cardinal clinical features are ophthalmoplegia with positive forced duction testing, visual loss, proptosis and pain. A Horner's syndrome has not yet been described secondary to a purely orbital lesion.

454. (F) Juvenile diabetics of long standing may present with hemorrhagic swelling of one or both discs with or without visual loss. Prognosis for return of vision is good, and invasive studies are not indicated.

455. (F) Recent evidence indicates the earliest detectable ophthalmoscopic change is swelling of the nerve fiber layer at the edge of the disc.

456. (F) In patients with pseudopapilledema, 68% of those with visible drusen and 21% of those without visible drusen have enlarged blind spots with formal field testing.

457. (F) An ascending optic atrophy model in the monkey indicates normal optic disc vasculature. Pallor seems to result from alterations in tissue reflectance and translucency following axonal loss and glial reorganization.

458. (T) Transient visual blurring following exercise in patients with optic neuritis is called Uhthoff's phenomenon, and is seen in up to 49% of patients.

459. (F) Unfortunately, attempts at surgical extirpation are not infrequently associated with dramatic loss of vision. Since these tumors are histologically benign and grow very slowly, conservative decompressive procedures or nonsurgical management are currently favored.

460. (T) Recent evidence indicates that brain stem neuronal outflow synapses also with small neurons in the abducens nucleus which travel to the opposite MLF and reach the contralateral medial rectus muscle.

461. (F) Clinical evidence indicates that ACTH treatment shortens the visual recovery time in patients with optic neuritis, but does not improve the final level of visual function when matched against a similar nontreated control group.

462. (F) The inferior branch of the oculomotor nerve supplies the inferior rectus, medial rectus, inferior oblique, pupil and ciliary body. The nerve branches as it enters the orbit, and posterior communicating aneurysms do not usually affect it selectively.

463. (F) Traumatic oculomotor palsy is usually seen with severe head trauma. When seen in association with minor head trauma, it may be indicative of prior subclinical dysfunction from an aneurysm or tumor, and requires further evaluation.

464. (F) One patient in six with bilateral tonic pupils has a positive serological test for syphilis.

465. (F) At times, slight to moderate atrophy may be associated with an excellent postoperative visual result. A horizontal band of thinning and atrophy of the retinal nerve fiber layer adjacent to the disc (secondary to retrograde axonal degeneration) more reliably predicts permanent field defects.

466. (F) Defective accommodation with blurred near vision especially when fatigued has been reported. Although pupillary abnormalities are not seen with routine clinical observation, pupillographic recordings demonstrate a reduced amplitude, velocity, and acceleration of pupillary constriction which is corrected by edrophonium.

467.   (T) Obstruction of orbital venous drainage at the level of the superior orbital fissure/anterior cavernous sinus is a frequent radiographic finding in the Tolosa-Hunt syndrome.

468.   (T) Varying degrees of pupillary inequality may be seen in up to 20% of the "normal" population, without pathological significance.

469.   (F) Childhood optic gliomas are static to slow growing glial hamartomas with a clinically benign course. Glioblastoma is the rule in adult onset optic gliomas with a downhill course to death in several months to two years.

470.   (T) Positional nystagmus from a peripheral source has a latent period of 3-40 seconds before becoming evident, habituates upon repeated testing and is poorly reproducible, with associated intense subjective vertigo. Central positional nystagmus may begin immediately, habituates poorly, is reproducible and is usually associated with mild subjective vertigo.

471.   (F) Congenital nystagmus is binocular, of similar amplitude in both eyes, always in the same plane in all fields of gaze, increased by attempts at fixation, and may be associated with head nodding although there is usually no oscillopsia. Latent nystagmus may be demonstrated, and a superimposed opticokinetic nystagmus may give a response opposite to that expected.

472.   (F) Seventy-five percent of optic nerve gliomas present in the first decade, and ninety percent within the first two decades of life.

473.   (F) In a series of 63 patients, involvement of the third order oculosympathetic neuron by tumor was rare, being seen in only one case. Involvement of the second order oculosympathetic neuron by tumor is much more frequent.

474.   (T) Contraction of the field is rare, with the defective field being totally blind to all stimuli. It indicates a lesion which is total in its effect on the usual pathway, stable or nonprogressive, and usually prognostically poor for recovery.

475.   (F) Conjunctival telangiectasias are a constant feature in this syndrome.

476. (F) Almost all pathological ocular oscillations diminish or disappear with sleep. Ocular myoclonus is one exception.

477. (F) Vestibular nystagmus is suppressed by fixation, and increased in amplitude in the dark or with eye closure.

478. (F) Both are characterized by mixed lymphocyte-plasma cell inflammation infiltrate within the orbit or superior orbital fissure, respectively.

479. (C) There is hyposomnia with marked decrease in REM sleep and abnormal non-REM sleep patterns.

480. (D) This finding was seen in the acute stage in 10 patients and disappeared with clinical improvement.

481. (E) This phenomenon is considered to be nonspecific and not even of increased frequency in epileptics.

482. (C) The fact that hypothermia can cause an electrocerebral silence is well known. In a recent report, the same thing was observed in hyperthermia.

483. (C) Alpha coma usually ends in death shortly thereafter. A small percentage of patients recover with residual cognitive deficits.

484. (A) Focal arrhythmic delta (often at 1Hz or less) is generally reported with brain abscesses. In a recent series, it was seen in 100%.

485. (C) This study indicated that larger heads tend to produce slower alpha rhythms. The alpha frequency also tends to be lower in subjects above age 60.

486. (B) This figure includes findings of uncertain significance but the incidence of clear abnormalities is higher than in asymptomatic persons.

487. (D) In a recent study, 71% of psychiatric patients had EEG abnormalities which were not expected from an abnormal neurologic history, exam, etc. Thus, it is appropriate for all psychiatric patients to have an EEG.

488. (D) Mu tends to shift sides normally but may be pathologic if consistently ipsilateral; ipsilateral disease was seen in 67% of a recent series of such cases.

489. (E) In a recent series, asynchronous sleep activity was seen 66% of the time with seizure discharges in 60%.

490. (A) The findings with subdural and subarachnoid hemorrhage are extremely variable, whereas epidural hematoma would more likely produce lateralized and projected slowing.

491. (D) Various relationships exist between alcohol and seizures. In a recent study, alcohol had an activating effect in a large majority of patients.

492. (E) Although it is commonly assumed that rage attacks are a form of complex partial seizures, this is almost never the cause as shown in a recent study.

493. (D) This EEG finding has been controversial since its initial description. Recent data show a highly significant correlation with certain forms of head trauma.

494. (A) Although PLED's are a nonspecific finding, authors agree that it is most commonly seen in vascular disease, especially CVA's.

495. (A) Although 14 and 6 are a controversial finding, the correlation with autonomic symptoms has been established for some time.

496. (C) 67% of patients in a recent study were confused but the range of consciousness was quite variable.

497. (C) Patients with supratentorial lesions usually have normal records; wave I is a far-field eighth nerve potential.

498. (C) The lesion in alpha coma is in the brain stem below the diencephalon. Thus, only visual cortical EP's are present; brain stem or "far field" A and SS EP's are usually present, however.

499. (A) While all choices except E may show seizure activity, sleep deprivation of 24 hours or more is most likely to be positive. This is often difficult to achieve.

500. (D) The first two changes relate to the direct damage of the biopsy. Choice C is related to the absence of skull over the biopsy site.

501. (B) In a recent study, 89% of patients with PA and associated mental dysfunction had abnormal EEG's.

502. (E) Choice A may be correct in some cases, but drug levels are more useful than the EEG for monitoring compliance. Choice B would apply only in the case of coma. Choice D is correct if A and B are ruled out.

503. (E) No definite prediction can be made although the findings in choices B and D increase the likelihood of seizure development.

504. (C) This well known but rare phenomenon was recently described in two patients, one with bilateral occipital sharp waves and no effect of photic stimulation, and the other with diffuse seizure discharges and a photoconvulsive response.

505. (B) EEG changes in dementia obviously depend on the stage of the disease. Therefore, a normal EEG does not rule out this diagnosis.

506. (B) The EEG and clinical findings in arteritis are as variable as the vascular involvement. Focal or multifocal involvement is most common.

507. (E) This corresponds to a high incidence of clinical deficits (enlarging head 61%, seizure 50%, retardation 53%) in a recent study.

508. (D) In a recent study of 203 epileptic children, 72% had focal sharp waves.

509. (E) The authors interpret these findings to mean that limbic damage produces psychosis.

510. (B) Diffuse neurologic deficits accompanying this syndrome may be the responsible factors producing the EEG changes.

511. (A) Seizures in this period are often benign. The lack of EEG seizure activity may reflect this. Definite or possible seizure discharges were found in 17% of a recent series of 6,723 cases.

512. (C) Much of the EEG slowing associated with tumors is related to edema and therefore promptly responds to dexamethasone according to a recent report. Choices A, B and D are nonspecific findings.

513.   (D) They must be differentiated from 14 and 6/sec. positive bursts and electrical artifacts. Most patients with focal positive spikes have convulsive disorders.

514.   (A) F-wave corresponds to the fastest motor nerve conduction velocity on the basis of this study and a review of the literature.

515.   (C) In one study, the neurologic status at age one was accurately predicted in 80% using all the above and 65% using the EEG alone.

516.   (E) Recording standards have been rigidly defined including all the choices plus others. Erroneous "false-positive" interpretations may result when these minimum technical standards are not adhered to.

517.   (D) There are typical myotonic responses but also spontaneous fibrillation and some myopathic abnormalities that are not seen in other forms of myotonia.

518.   (B) Recovery has been described in drug (including anesthetic) overdose. Accordingly, cerebral death should not be diagnosed on the basis of a single examination if there is any suspicion of drug overdose.

519.   (A) Diffuse slow rhythms also occur but the photic stimulation response is most striking (photoconvulsive or photomyoclonic response often resulting in clinical seizures).

520.   (D) The characteristic EEG pattern is known as hypsarrhythmia. This EEG term is often applied to the clinical attacks.

521.   (B) Around 50% of patients have abnormal EEG's of various nonspecific types. The EEG findings alone seldom suggest the diagnosis, seldom directly reflect plaques and seldom consist of seizure discharges.

522.   (A) While answers B through E are possibilities, such a picture is consistent with a healing infarction. In the presence of clinical improvement, diagnosis of a new lesion becomes tenuous. Serial EEG's may be indicated.

523.   (E) Tegmental (reticular) pathways are preserved in this state so that consciousness (and EEG patterns) are unaffected.

524. (D) In childhood, there may be a significant discrepancy between the degree of trauma and the EEG. Serial tracings help to establish the nature of the findings.

525. (D) There is a general correlation of the state of consciousness (but not the creatinine, BUN, etc.) and the EEG. In general, the slower the EEG the more comatose the patient.

526. (D) While bilaterally synchronous, frontally dominant triphasic waves suggest metabolic disease; the diagnosis depends on the total clinical and laboratory picture.

527. (E) The vasculitis of this disease may be focal, multifocal or diffuse. Accordingly, the EEG findings are just as variable.

528. (C) This relatively high incidence of abnormalities has been variously accounted for by postulating latent epilepsy, immaturity and limbic lesions.

529. (D) REM sleep correlates best with nocturnal migraine.

530. (C) Even though clinical seizures occur in these situations, diffuse slowing only occurred in one series.

531. (E) EEG changes may be found but the incidence of these is no different than in the average population. Therefore, EEG abnormalities in this setting suggest another etiology.

532. (C) Recovery does not occur from the first two choices. "Alpha coma" usually implies a poor prognosis. Recovery from a state of low voltage delta certainly can occur but no predictive statements can be made.

533. (D) There is generally a marked midline shift so that the EEG is always abnormal. The shift generally affects diencephalic structures to the extent that lateralized findings are obscured in favor of diffuse abnormalities.

534. (E) Choices A through C represent nonspecific findings which do not suggest a diagnosis. In all likelihood, the EEG will not be normal. Periodic abnormalities are seen in several clinical states but in this clinical setting strongly suggest the diagnosis.

535.   (A) The EEG in dementing disease is usually nonspecific; careful interpretation of "soft" EEG signs may be of some assistance.

536.   (D) It behaves in a passive discharging manner.

537.   (D) These EMG potentials are considered fairly specific for this disease.

538.   (A) In patients with periodic paralysis, usually during an attack there is complete electrical silence.

539.   (A) This is most consistent with this condition.

540.   (A) This neurodiagnostic test can reveal a disturbed neuromuscular function even in the absence of clinical symptoms by detecting an increased jitter.

541.   (C) Choices A and B should produce lateralized slowing which more often is irregular. The EEG in delirium tremens is generally normal.

542.   (E) There is a close correspondence of reticular function and the EEG. In choices A through D, coma results from reticular dysfunction.

543.   (D) These electrodes reflect mesial temporal discharges which are detected by scalp electrodes in the vast majority of cases. They are prone to various artefacts which can mimic seizure discharge. They are often uncomfortable and, therefore, prevent sleep, the most valuable activating procedure. Their use is indicated, however, in patients with suspected temporal lobe epilepsy and a previously normal sleep EEG.

544.   (B) Meningitis and encephalitis would normally cause diffuse slowing. Focal slowing may occur with a tumor or an abscess but tumors are usually associated with considerable edema affecting adjacent areas.

545.   (D) The basic frequency of the EEG correlates with the stage of the disease. Therefore, alpha of 8 Hz (with the usual frequency being 10 Hz) may be significant. The diagnosis is neither confirmed nor ruled out.

546.   (D) Biochemical changes with the exception of serum ammonia do not correlate with the EEG changes and the correlation is too general to be of use in the individual

patient. The EEG is a sensitive indicator of changes in consciousness, however.

547. (B) While triphasic waves are nonspecific, when focal they often suggest focal disease.

548. (A) The EEG is rather specific for this diagnosis in the setting of a presenile dementia. The diagnosis is confirmed further if the triphasic waves correlate with myoclonic jerks.

549. (D) This type of change is only seen in demyelinating diseases.

550. (E) The small yield must be considered in the light of these considerations and the considerable technical difficulties of obtaining adequate deprivation.

551. (C) Such bursts may be associated with seizure discharges, or seizure activity may be represented by slow activity in scalp leads. However, they occur in many other disorders and, therefore, are nonspecific.

552. (A) The findings correlate respectively with central necrosis and peripheral gliosis. This pathologic combination is common in neoplasia.

553. (E) Changes occur in white matter diseases such as Tay-Sachs, but these are usually pseudoperiodic and consist of triphasic waves. Strictly periodic sharp-slow bursts are nearly specific for SSPE in a child. The interburst interval is also longer.

554. (A) This finding is recognized as a normal age change. The disease in the other choices could also be responsible, however, and further workup is advisable.

555. (C) Lesions must affect cortical or ascending reticular fibers to cause changes. Since the lateral medullary area (the site of the lesion in Wallenberg's) does not contain such fibers, the EEG is normal.

556. (D) Because of the bad prognosis associated with suppression bursts, choices A and C should be ruled out before suppression burst is interpreted.

557. (D) Intrinsic cerebral activity is usually of normal form and distribution during waking and sleep periods.

558. (A) In prematures, trace alternant is the dominant EEG rhythm. It consists of short sequences of moderate amplitude, very slow waves alternating with low-amplitude, poorly defined activity.

559. (C) Answer D may be correct but mild hypoglycemia may be the etiology of the finding. This should be ruled out before the EEG is interpreted as abnormal.

560. (D) The findings could all be secondary to the surgery. Only if the slowing is more extensive than the surgical area, or if the slowing is progressive on serial EEG's can the EEG be said to suggest recurrence.

561. (B) The effect of the bone is attenuation and filtering of faster EEG rhythms. Thus, the EEG is abnormal, but only indicates a lack of bone. Answers C and D would be possible if there were some abnormal slowing as well.

562. (C) The finding is regarded as nonepileptic by most authorities, because clinical seizures are not associated with it. However, it is not felt to be normal and does have associated clinical problems.

563. (E) Possibly the most important association is with drug usage so that the occurrence of this finding in a diffusely slow EEG may point to drugs as an etiology for the slowing.

564. (A) Both early and late SSEP components are lost or decreased over the contralateral hemispheres whereas the EEG in a recent series was frequently normal or diffusely slow.

565. (A) Numerous studies have shown that two types of Charcot-Marie-Tooth disease exist; the hypertrophic (demyelinating) and the neuronal (loss of large myelinated fibers).

566. (B) The amygdala also shows high acetylcholinesterase activity.

567. (C) While the finding of EEG slowing may occur with either situation, the frequency of the slowing tends to be less with hypercalcemia.

568. (A) Dramatic and prompt improvement in the EEG is the rule with treatment.

569. (B) Even minimal decreases below normal of the blood sugar may cause EEG changes. These rapidly disappear with rising glucose levels.

570. (B) They range from 1-150 Hz at 10-300 microvolt amplitude.

571. (A) The other conditions can be distinguished from rum fits by abnormal interictal EEG's and historical information.

572. (A) Focal slowing as well as focal spikes or spike-waves do occur. Mild, intermittent slow activity may be seen in symptom-free patients.

573. (D) "Silent" areas with respect to the EEG are present including the internal capsule and the basal portion of the brain stem. Choice B is incorrect, however, because brain stem lesions would not cause aphasia.

574. (B) While choice D is theoretically rational, the right-to-left frequency gradient suggests a right-sided lesion. Moreover, the EEG can be a sensitive index of edema, a potentially dangerous situation. A CT scan should be obtained.

575. (C) They are related to myelination.

576. (A) If the cell membrane potential is reduced by an applied voltage stimulus, sodium ions will enter the cell at an increasing rate, thereby reducing still further the membrane potential. The nature of this self-generating mechanism involved in the development of the action potential was delineated by Hodgkin and Huxley in 1952.

577. (A) The only reports to the contrary were in the 1950s without adequate control of the now known variables.

578. (C) This is a genetically determined condition and values are consistent within families.

579. (B) It is normal or very mildly slowed in the axonal degeneration type of neuropathy.

580. (C) These electrographic findings may be helpful in diagnosis of these cerebromacular degeneration states.

581. (B) Same as 580.

582.   (A) Same as 580.

583.   (T) This relates to delayed or incomplete transmission.

584.   (T) Both destructive processes may produce irregular polymorphic slow delta waves.

585.   (F) Significant pathology (i.e. meningiomas or subdural hematomas) may occur with normal EEG patterns.

586.   (F) It is inversely proportional to internodal spacing, i.e. the longer the internodal spacing the less current required to reach threshold.

587.   (T) This is the node to node conduction (saltatory conduction) concept.

588.   (T) Larger diameter fibers conduct faster.

589.   (F) Indirectly related; i.e. the larger the diameter, the smaller the internal resistance.

590.   (T) The various fibers which constitute the nerve differ in their level of excitability.

591.   (F) Primarily the sodium ion via the sodium pump.

592.   (F) Saltatory conduction is characteristic of myelinated nerve fibers.

593.   (C) Meningiomas are more often oval in shape, being round in less than one-third of the cases, whereas acoustic neuromas are characteristically round (over 90% of cases).

594.   (D) All are correct. Dyke, Davidoff and Masson first described radiographic findings of cerebral hemiatrophy usually due to an acute episode of brain trauma or infection at birth or in early childhood.

595.   (A) In a series of 349 CT scans performed for possible orbital abnormalities, scleral thickening with contrast enhancement was found in 50% of the cases of orbital pseudotumor.

596.   (A) Hypoplasias are not features of arachnoid cysts but are part of the Dandy-Walker syndrome. Answers B, C and D are common to both entities.

597.   (E) The risk of serious complication becomes greater
        as catheterization of a vessel becomes more difficult.
        Left vertebral artery catheterization produced fewest
        complications of any of the four vessels in this and other
        studies.

598.   (C) All except the malformations are not infrequently
        present with lupus.

599.   (D) There appear to be few false-positives with various
        atrophic diseases of the central nervous system using a
        CT scan frontal horn/bicaudate ratio of less than 1.6 as
        the criterion.

600.   (E) Similar changes appear with malignant tumors and
        differentiation may be impossible.

601.   (D) CT was more reliable than angiography in this series
        in determining which one of multiple aneurysms had bled.

602.   (C) Hydrocephalus is more frequent with craniopharyn-
        gioma (10/17 cases) than with pituitary adenomas (3/26
        cases).

603.   (D) In all patients with normal contrast and noncontrast
        CT scans using multiple cut technique, further evaluation
        of the suprasellar region by angiography or pneumoen-
        cephalography proved unrewarding.

604.   (B) In a series of 8,500 CT scans with 65 proven para-
        sellar masses, hypothalamic glioma was less common
        than the other four choices listed.

605.   (A) Approximately 30% of patients with moderate or se-
        vere signs and symptoms of M.S. have plaques demon-
        strable by CT.

606.   (E) Excessive dilution of the amipaque contrast column
        becomes a problem during complete myelograms since
        the time required for careful fluoroscopy and film studies
        is necessarily increased.

607.   (E) Convexity metrizamide is visualized as a cortical
        stain on conventional CT cisternograms. Until coronal
        CT imaging is improved, the CSF flow over the convexi-
        ties is best visualized by radionuclide cisternograms.

608. (A) Such scan findings in a child with this history should suggest the diagnosis.

609. (D) The opposite is the case, i. e. recurrence was more frequent in the lytic group as opposed to those presenting with hyperostotic changes.

610. (B) A peripheral contusion may present as a rim of slightly higher density than adjacent brain next to the inner table of the skull, and is often difficult to distinguish from a small extracerebral collection.

611. (D) Cerebral edema was an acute CT finding observed within the first week following trauma in 37 to 45 scans reviewed. It did not occur after 6 weeks.

612. (C) Capillary hemangioma is independent of the optic nerve although large lesions may obscure it. Only optic nerve gliomas and meningiomas produce enlarged optic nerves on CT.

613. (D) Computerized tomography proved insensitive to leptomeningeal spread of hematologic malignancies including leukemia, lymphoma and malignant histiocytosis.

614. (B) This portion of the nerve is not clearly demonstrated because of the bony density of the canal and the proximity of muscle tendons.

615. (E) The association of a large supratentorial mass with considerable shift of midline structures and CT findings of a dilated contralateral temporal horn should be considered indicative of tentorial herniation.

616. (A) Although the decrease in brain volume may in part be secondary to steroid-induced protein catabolism, other mechanisms appear to be operative as well, including changes in vascular permeability, water and sodium diuresis, loss of brain water, and the effects of the underlying disease process itself.

617. (C) Dilatation of the lateral ventricles of moderate or severe degree is present in the majority of cerebellar tumors.

618. (A) The brain has a limited response to pathologic lesions. The presence of edema and mass effect may indicate brain tumor or cerebral infarction.

619. (B) Specific localization to a given lobe of the brain may be difficult with CT, and therefore the surgeon may desire a radionuclide scan in addition to CT for more confident localization.

620. (E) A defect in the lambdoid suture just posterior to the junction of the parietomastoid and the occipitomastoid suture is commonly seen in neurofibromatosis.

621. (B) Multiple sclerosis plaques do not typically calcify.

622. (E) Although CT has largely replaced air encephalography for initial investigation of children with hydrocephalus, several conditions require pneumoencephalography supplemented by polytomography for accurate analysis including those listed.

623. (E) Multi-infarct dementia, in addition to generalized atrophy, often has more focal components, i.e. large cortical lucent defects.

624. (C) The most common area of white matter involvement is in the occipital or occipitoparietal portions of the cerebral hemispheres.

625. (B) While platybasia may accompany basilar impression, it is not always present.

626. (B) Only 5% of these tumors are denser than surrounding brain on routine CT scan.

627. (E) All are true.

628. (D) In cases where the cyst wall does not blush after contrast, it most frequently represents benign reactive host tissue. When the cyst wall does blush after contrast, it is frequently found to contain tumor cells and probably represents degeneration of initially solid neoplasm.

629. (D) A well-defined "rim sign" is indicative of a later phase when the area of cerebritis has become encapsulated and liquefaction of the center has occurred.

630. (B) Patterns of enhancement with infarction are variable and nonspecific and may simulate other entities such as brain tumor, inflammatory lesions, and especially AVM.

631. (E) The ring blush is a definite stage in the evolution of an aging hematoma, and does not necessarily indicate underlying neoplasm or supervening abscess.

632. (A) The response of the brain and meninges to differing disease processes is limited, thus the appearance of inflammatory lesions on CT may be similar to many other pathologic processes.

633. (A) Chronic subdural hematomas are often D-shaped or crescentic.

634. (D) All are correct.

635. (E) Computed tomography is altering the significance of ventriculography and is the initial procedure of choice for identifying presence of hydrocephalus and obstructing lesions producing it.

636. (B) For mass lesions suspected of being in the cerebral hemispheres with or without hydrocephalus, computed tomography and angiography are the procedures of choice.

637. (E) Dandy-Walker and arachnoid cysts may be confused angiographically. Initial computerized tomography scan and subsequent air studies best identify these lesions.

638. (A) Mucopolysaccharidoses produce metabolic megalencephaly due to intracellular accumulations of abnormal metabolic products.

639. (B) Meningeal vessels may also supply other extracerebral tumors including neurinomas, hemangioblastomas, chordomas and tumors of nasopharynx. When intracerebral tumors such as glioblastoma invade the dura, meningeal vessels may contribute to their supply.

640. (C) Early venous filling is certainly not a pathognomonic sign, but may be seen in many varied clinical conditions.

641. (B) Epidural venography is more accurate than myelography at L5-S1 and with lateral herniations.

642. (C) They are typical of an intradural, extramedullary lesion.

643. (D) The normal diameter of the internal auditory canal ranges from 2 to 10 mm with a mean of 5.0 mm.

644. (B) Meningitis is more prone to cause a block in infancy.

645. (D) The meningeal branches of the internal maxillary artery are the most common sources of the shunt in cases of external carotid cavernous sinus fistula; middle meningeal and ascending pharyngeal arteries are also frequent sources.

646. (C) The empty sella is quite common in subjects with slow-growing hormone producing tumors, especially those accompanied by acromegaly, but there is no increased occurrence with chromophobe adenomas. Increased incidence of empty sella occurs with conditions A and D also.

647. (C) The lateral ventricles are dilated in these small children. Subdural collections may interfere with CSF absorption thereby producing ventricular dilatation as well as prominent sulci and fissures.

648. (C) Usually, the tumor blush is intense and nearly homogeneous. No medulloblastoma had a ring blush in the series quoted.

649. (B) Tonsillar herniation is not conclusively identified without prior introduction of intrathecal metrizamide.

650. (D) Four patterns of abnormal curves were recognized in this study, and it is believed these patterns help to characterize different lesions.

651. (A) In contrast to the much more common epidural abscess, osteomyelitis is not associated with spinal subdural abscess.

652. (D) It is safe to selectively catheterize this artery when studying patients for possible AVM for example. After contrast injection, the vessel is flushed with physiologic saline and the catheter is removed at once.

653. (B) Drainage into deep central veins is common.

654. (T) Repeated poorly controlled seizures which require large doses of multiple anticonvulsant drugs probably account for these findings.

655. (C) Mercury attacks the neuron cell body preferentially, the others attack the axon initially.

656.   (C) Specific toxins to the acetylcholine receptor site provided the big breakthrough which was supported by electron microscopic studies and animal models.

657.   (D) Previously thought to be necessarily absent for a "brain death" diagnosis, this reflex merely indicates peripheral sympathetic intactness.

658.   (A) Most studies show amantadine effect to peak very early and fall off by several months to a year. A definite withdrawal effect occurs upon acute discontinuation.

659.   (A) GABA is lowered in CSF as well; the decarboxylase is low compared to normal brain tissues.

660.   (D) It is commonly assumed that an EEG drug effect is increased beta. In actual fact, only a few categories of drugs have this effect as a major one.

661.   (C) Application of drugs that either antagonize or mimic the effects of GABA on central neurons produced wave-spike seizures. Hence, petit mal epilepsy could result from dysfunction of GABA-ergic neurons.

662.   (D) All are dopamine agonists.

663.   (D) All drugs listed are involved in the alteration of serotonin levels.

664.   (C) The catecholamine, dopamine, is involved in Parkinson's disease; the enzymes related to the synthesis and degradation of dopamine are also involved.

665.   (B) The restoration of presynaptic inhibition prevents the spread of electrical discharges from the epileptic focus to the rest of the brain.

666.   (D) Conversion of the amino acid tyrosine to DOPA is the rate limiting step in the biosynthesis of catecholamines, and the synthesis is dependent on the activity of tyrosine hydroxylase.

667.   (A) The endogenous transmitter is blocked.

668.   (B) PAM removes the phosphate group from the phosphorylated enzyme resulting from the formation of a complex between the enzyme and organophosphate compounds.

669. (E) The major catabolic pathway for histidine proceeds via urocanic acid, formiminoglutamic acid and glutamic acid. Histidinemia is the result of an interruption in the first step of the pathway because of a defect in histidase.

670. (B) Pompe's disease is glycogen storage disease type II and is characterized by glycogen accumulation in skeletal muscles, heart, liver and central nervous system.

671. (D) The vertebral arteries provide segmental arteries for the cervical cord, aortic segmentals supply the thoracic and lumbar cord.

672. (A) Transketolase requires thiamine pyrophosphate as a co-factor, and using TPP as an activator gives specificity to the assay.

673. (A) Infantile Gaucher's disease (cerebroside lipidosis) is the result of almost complete absence of glucocerebrosidase with an excess of glucocerebroside in the liver and spleen.

674. (C) It is the result of a defect of lipid-transporting peptides. This is a rare disorder associated with cerebellar and posterior column signs, retinal degeneration and acanthocytosis.

675. (A) The anterior 1/3 of the optic tract receives twigs from the internal carotid, middle cerebral, and posterior communicating arteries. The posterior 2/3 is supplied by the anterior choroidal artery.

676. (D) In patients suffering from parkinsonism, the dopamine levels are markedly decreased. Administration of L-dopa, the precursor for dopamine synthesis, elevates the dopamine levels.

677. (A) In cases of malignant hyperpyrexia, calcium in the muscle sarcoplasmic reticulum has been found to be increased. Its significance needs further study.

678. (D) All can produce myotonia in humans.

679. (D) Although almost never found without iatrogenic intervention, phosphorus depletion is most commonly seen in chronic alcoholics, treated diabetic acidosis and hyperalimentation.

680.   (B) This most commonly occurs in renal failure and, if severe, may cause total paralysis and cardiac arrest.

681.   (D) These manifestations are identical with hypertensive encephalopathy, sometimes with a superimposed intra-cerebral hematoma.

682.   (D) Ataxia is related to blood levels and does not con-stitute a contraindication to continued use. Erythema multiforme, hepatitis and Stevens-Johnson syndrome are evidence of hypersensitivity and are absolute contrain-dications to further use of the drug.

683.   (E) Enhancement occurs with drugs that deplete endog-enous catecholamines or block the catecholaminergic receptors.

684.   (E) All are possible.

685.   (E) All may cause it.

686.   (B) Inhibition of acetylcholinesterase is to prevent the hydrolysis of acetylcholine. When acetylcholine is not re-leased in denervated organs, no pharmacological response is seen.

687.   (C) Dopa exists in carboxylated form and dopa decar-boxylase cleaves the COOH group; pyridoxal phosphate is an essential co-factor for this reaction.

688.   (C) Such a high rate of oxygen consumption is required because the brain is the most metabolically active organ in the body.

689.   (B) These occur in nearly 20%. The misinnervation usually involves the median and ulnar nerves and leads to confusion on clinical examination.

690.   (A) Almost all patients will excrete twice as much as normals. This, along with low serum ceruloplasmin con-centration and detection of Kayser-Fleischer rings con-stitute good tests for this disease.

691.   (B) The reason for this change is not clear at present, but the decrease was significant.

692.   (B) Only HVA is elevated; this may reflect cerebral is-chemia and release of vasoactive amines.

693. (C) Maximal induced hyperpolarization occurs at the potassium equilibrium potential with no involvement of the electrogenic sodium pump.

694. (C) Both are capable of destroying acetylcholine. However, the location of acetylcholinesterase is at the transmission site, whereas the pseudocholinesterase is found in plasma.

695. (T) Inhibition of dopamine action at the receptor site by blockade with phenothiazine drugs may produce parkinsonism.

696. (T) All these processes consume relatively high amounts of energy.

697. (F) Cerebral metabolism is not decreased during sleep.

698. (T) The loss or low level of lipids is the characteristic feature of demyelination.

699. (F) When myelin is lost, extracellular fluid, astrocytes and inflammatory cells accumulate and these are more hydrated than myelin.

700. (T) All portions of these statements are correct.

701. (T) The levels of these metabolites are measured in order to assess the turnover of dopamine in patients.

702. (F) These drugs increase the turnover of dopamine and may produce an increase in homovanillic acid in CSF.

703. (T) Catecholamines such as dopamine and norepinephrine are well known neurotransmitters having various central functions.

704. (T) Conclusive evidence is not available, but various reports have shown altered levels of this important inhibitory neurotransmitter in these diseases.

705. (T) Toxicity to diphenylhydantoin develops in 10% of patients on therapeutic doses of the drug who are then placed on isoniazid.

706. (T) Refsum's disease is a disease of phytanic acid metabolism.

707. (T) The secondary amines produce psychomotor agitation and have less affinity for alpha-noradrenergic binding sites.

708. (C) The two naturally occurring alkaloids exert actions similar to acetylcholine.

709. (D) These enzymes are abnormal or deficient in these conditions (709-713).

710. E
711. B
712. C
713. A
714. E
715. C
716. B
717. A
718. D
719. D

720. (T) Four out of 25 patients on valproate showed hepatic side effects; three of these showed reversal of these effects when valproic acid was reduced by 10 mg/kg per day.

721. (T) Neuropathological evidence indicates a loss of cerebellar climbing fibers in this disorder, and it may be that aspartic acid is the neurotransmitter of climbing fibers.

722. (F) The data show that phenytoin binds to albumin at a site different from valproic acid. Hence, phenytoin has no effect on valproic acid binding to albumin.

723. (T) Valproic acid structurally resembles free fatty acids having short carbon chains and both may have affinity for the same site on the albumin, resulting in an increased binding of valproic acid.

724. (F) The biological half-life of sodium valproate is 6-9 hours; it is known to peak in serum within 1-3 hours after an oral dose.

725. (F) The transfer of phenobarbital from plasma to saliva is greatly influenced by the pH of saliva.

726. (T) The data suggest that the decrease in beta-adrenergic receptor binding in aged human cerebellum is due to a reduction in the number of receptor sites rather than a change in affinity, which means it is related to cell loss with age.

727. (T) Decamethonium, choline, and acetylcholine do not have their normal depolarizing action in myasthenic patients; instead, they produce a curare-type competitive block. These findings point to a postjunctional change probably involving receptor sites.

728. (T) The frequency of the miniature end plate potentials is controlled by the conditions of the presynaptic membrane, while their amplitude is usually controlled by the postsynaptic element.

729. (T) This may be due to altered calcium metabolism in the dystrophic condition.

730. (F) It is known that convulsions produced by 100% oxygen could be prevented by antioxidants. Vitamin E administration in this study showed a decreased seizure production.

731. (T) It can be blocked by application of scopolamine in the cat.

732. (T) The ratio of plasma glycine to CSF glycine provides evidence that the glycine cleavage enzymes are defective in the brain. The ratio is greatly reduced from the normal value of 35.

733. (F) This is unlikely, and, in fact, the status of the disease as an entity is in doubt.

734. (F) Vasogenic edema confined to the white matter is associated with brain tumors.

735. (T) Acetylcholine, as well as choline acetyl transferase, the enzyme necessary for its production, are both reduced.

736. (T) This is the abnormality.

737. (C) In a fetus with MLD, sulfatide accumulation was found in Schwann cells prior to myelination and early myelination elsewhere appeared normal. At least in the early stages, sulfatide storage appears to be distinct from the leukodystrophy which develops later.

738. (C) Golgi preparations suggest that microgyria results from a pathologic process operating on midcortical regions in a basically intact 6-layered cortex. This apparently occurs after cellular migrations are essentially complete and before secondary gyri develop, which is about the sixth month.

739. (D) Pituitary microadenomas, which may not be evident even on polytomography, are probably much more common than formerly realized and are amenable to transsphenoidal resection.

740. (A) Most recorded instances of radiation myelopathy have occurred when unconventional fractionation schemes have been used.

741. (B) 101 ependymomas were the object of this study; glioblastomas are far more common lesions.

742. (E) Hemorrhage does not seem to play a role.

743. (D) All are true.

744. (E) Tuberous sclerosis usually appears in childhood or adult life. 13 cases occurring during the first week of life have been reported.

745. (E) It is easy to single out venous thrombosis as the main cause of cerebral white matter hemorrhagic necrosis; however, systemic factors also play an important role.

746. (C) There is marked hypotonia.

747. (B) In Wernicke's encephalopathy, the mamillary bodies are involved in most cases (91-95%), but not in SNEM.

748. (D) There is a high degree of vulnerability of human fetal brain to maternal intoxication by methyl mercury. The major defect appears to be related to faulty development and not to focal neuronal damage as observed in mercury intoxication in adults and children exposed postnatally.

749. (D) In an examination of three brains showing fibrinoid degeneration and miliary aneurysm formation in the arterioles, two of the patients had not been clinically hypertensive.

750.   (D) All are correct.

751.   (B) Thymic germinal center hyperplasia is present in
       65% of cases of MG.

752.   (C) It is about 1/8th as common as intraspinal tumors,
       most common between ages 40 and 60, and is pathologi-
       cally a diffuse opacification and thickening of the arach-
       noidal membranes.

753.   (A) In Friedreich's ataxia, the predominant abnormality
       in peripheral nerve fibers is a decreased number of large
       myelinated fibers.

754.   (E) The pathological features of Menkes disease include
       neuronal loss and myelin depletion, but one of the strik-
       ing features is severe atrophy of the granular layer of
       the cerebellar cortex.

755.   (A) A deficiency or abnormality of peroxisomes has been
       described in two disorders, the cerebrohepatorenal syn-
       drome and acatalasemia.

756.   (B) Segmental distention of axons (giant axonal neurop-
       athy) is the principal neuropathic feature of n-hexane
       toxicity. Although there is little demyelination, electro-
       diagnostic findings paradoxically are those of demyelina-
       tive neuropathy.

757.   (C) Endothelial proliferation is more typical of gliomas.
       The rest are common in metastatic tumors.

758.   (E) There is loss of dendritic spines with progressive
       deterioration of the elements of the dendritic domain.

759.   (E) Trophoblastic tissue penetrates and proliferates in
       vascular tissue, and may result in any of these lesions.

760.   (B) Although suprasellar cysts are common, an enlarged
       temporal fossa with an atrophic anterior temporal tip oc-
       cupied by a large cyst is most common.

761.   (D) Cysts in the posterior fossa arising elsewhere than
       the vermis, although they occur, are very rare; mid-
       line cysts often extend up through the incisura.

762. (A) The clinical feature that is characteristic of status marmoratus is choreoathetosis.

763. (D) Together, neurofibromas and meningiomas constitute 55% of all intraspinal tumors.

764. (C) Descriptive of their peculiar histologic staining reaction, ragged red fibers are muscle fibers which contain abnormal mitochondria. They are most consistently found in the Kearns-Sayre syndrome, in which CSF immunoglobulins are usually elevated.

765. (D) One breakdown of primary sites as percentages of all metastatic tumor is: lung, 35%; breast, 20%, skin (melanoma), 5-10%; kidney, 5%

766. (A) Acrylamide has been useful experimentally because of the almost pure axonal degeneration it produces. The neuropathies produced by the other agents are largely demyelinative in type.

767. (A) Invasion of nerve roots by astrocytes, apparently derived from subpial regions of the spinal cord, is a consistent feature of Werdnig-Hoffmann disease. The question of whether the disease is primarily a radiculopathy remains unresolved.

768. (B) Brain lesions containing foamy histiocytes with PAS positive granules and bacillary bodies typical of Whipple's disease were found in a patient who had sleep disturbance, memory loss and ophthalmoplegia but no GI tract symptoms.

769. (A) In Wolman's disease (which is probably a lysosomal acid lipase deficiency), lipid droplets accumulate in the glia, nerve sheath cells, and parenchymal cells of visceral organs. Mental deterioration is usually evident within a few weeks of age.

770. (D) Tangier disease is a rare familial disorder. The characteristic lipid abnormality is a profound deficiency of plasma high density lipoproteins and accumulation of cholesterol esters in many tissues, and a neuropathy. The diagnosis is suggested by the increased size and peculiar yellow-orange coloration of the pharyngeal tonsils.

771. (E) This lesion occurs in early childhood; its course is rapid (average 6 months).

772.   (E) All may show this abnormality.

773.   (A) These elements worsen the prognosis.

774.   (A) The oligosaccharides accumulate.

775.   (C) Both may produce it.

776.   (D) This study supports that in the injured brain, in addition to the proliferation of endogeneous cells, there is evidence that mononuclear cells from the blood enter the injured nerve tissue.

777.   (C) Polyribosomes serve as sites for protein synthesis both in intact cells and in sedimented, cell free in vitro systems.

778.   (C) Only 18 cases have been reported in the literature, the majority associated with infantile hemiplegia.

779.   (T) This phenomenon, characterized by apathy, confusion, irritability and sometimes agitation, occurs 2-21 days after the insult and may lead to death.

780.   (F) Hypertrophy of Alzheimer type II astrocytes is the predominant change.

781.   (T) 40-70% occur in the frontal lobes.

782.   (F) They are remnants of the notochord and occur most often along the clivus and in the sacrococcygeal area.

783.   (F) In most series, neurofibromas and meningiomas are the most common type.

784.   (F) In fact, the microscopic picture is indistinguishable from that of multiple sclerosis.

785.   (T) In 20 patients with GM, examination of the spinal cord revealed leptomeningeal metastases in 5.

786.   (T) 25 cases of cranial nerve palsy secondary to radiotherapy are reported in this paper.

787.   (F) This report provides direct evidence that neuroblastoma cells circulate and can be recovered from peripheral blood of affected patients.

788. (T) The 5-year survival is unchanged by this treatment.

789. (T) It improved to some extent.

790. (T) Its damage is more proximal than that of many neurotoxic agents.

791. (T) The cell, unable to produce sufficient protein to maintain its metabolism, will atrophy and die.

792. (F) A study of 16, 311 primary CNS tumors revealed these lesions to be more common in blacks.

793. (T) A study of 16, 311 primary CNS tumors revealed these differences.

794. (T) Same as 793.
795. (T) Same as 793.
796. (F) Same as 793.

797. (T) It may occur after all of them.

798. (T) The most consistent pathological feature of the hypoxic premature is periventricular leukomalacia (white spots).

799. (F) Status marmoratus is a pathologic state primarily in the basal ganglia of children who suffered hypoxic-ischemic injury in the first two years of life. The insult is usually in the perinatal period.

800. (T) Ulegyria is an acquired lesion resulting in small sclerotic gyri.

801. (T) It is reported to have occurred in 9. 3% of 75 cases studied.

802. (T) Naegleria is a free-living ameba which is pathogenic for man. Infection, often acquired from swimming pools, usually occurs in younger individuals and produces a fulminant necrotizing meningoencephalitis. Another ameba, Acanthamoeba, typically causes a more chronic granulomatous encephalitis in older persons.

803. (T) Electron microscopy of muscle in Kuf's disease may show diagnostic subsarcolemmal collections of membrane bound inclusions containing characteristic curvilinear profiles.

804. (F) According to the authors, this event is very rare and only 9 cases are known in the world's literature.

805. (T) Metastases occur in the middle cerebral artery territory more frequently than in other vascular distributions. Tumors from the common primary sites, e. g., lung, breast, tend to be multiple.

806. (F) When the relative masses of the spinal cord and brain are considered, astrocytomas are approximately equally common in both structures.

807. (T) Microtubules have been found to be a very important neural subcellular structure in axoplasmic flow and axonal sprouting.

808. (T) In various embryological studies, it was found that Schwann cells originate from the neural crest.

809. (T) Experimental vasospasm produced in monkey cerebral arteries by subarachnoid hemorrhage supports this statement.

810. (T) The Purkinje dendritic system is highly sensitive to the aging process.

811. (F) The trigeminal artery, a part of the blood supply to the brain stem in early embryonic life and normally absorbed into the formation of the basilar artery, may persist as an anomalous, carotid-basilar anastomosis with an incidence of 1-2%, and can be the site of aneurysms or vascular malformations.

FOR EACH OF THE FOLLOWING MULTIPLE CHOICE QUES-
TIONS, SELECT THE ONE MOST APPROPRIATE ANSWER.

1. Multiple sclerosis is
   A. probably "acquired" long before it becomes symptomatic
   B. caused by a virus recoverable from plaques
   C. more common in Louisiana than in Minnesota
   D. all of these
   E. none of these

2. Tic douloureux responds least to
   A. carbamazepine
   B. phenytoin
   C. vasoconstrictors
   D. nerve avulsion
   E. intracranial nerve section

3. The prognosis of amyotrophic lateral sclerosis
   A. carries an overall 5-year survival of 10%
   B. carries an overall 5-year survival of 20%
   C. carries an overall 5-year survival of 80%
   D. is best in those whose disease begins after age 60
   E. none of these

4. Which is not characteristic of Melkersson-Rosenthal
   syndrome?
   A. Furrowed tongue
   B. Hypertension
   C. Recurrent facial paralyses
   D. Edema of the face
   E. Edema of the lips

5. Risk for development of future difficulties following the first febrile seizure is <u>least</u> in which group?
   A. Children with complex febrile seizures
   B. Children who have a family history of afebrile seizures
   C. Children who demonstrate abnormal neurologic function
   D. Children whose first febrile seizure occurs after age 2
   E. Children whose first febrile seizure occurs before 18 months of age

6. Childhood aphasia
   A. is more likely to recover if the insult occurs after age 6
   B. is usually fluent in kind
   C. is "crossed" much more frequently than in adults
   D. occurs after left hemisphere lesions in 90-95% of cases
   E. none of these

7. Refsum's disease is characterized by all the following except
   A. nerve deafness
   B. autosomal dominant transmission usually
   C. it is most common in Caucasians
   D. retinitis pigmentosa
   E. ataxia

8. Hand preference is not usually developed until
   A. 5 months
   B. 8 months
   C. 11 months
   D. 14 months
   E. 18 months

9. A reflex not usually present until age 10 months is the
   A. Palmar grasp
   B. Landau
   C. Moro
   D. Rooting
   E. Plantar grasp

10. Myasthenia in children
    A. is not associated with thyrotoxicosis
    B. is associated with thyrotoxicosis in 50%
    C. is associated with poor response to medication and an irreversible course in 10-20%
    D. is far more common in males than in females
    E. usually begins before age 2

11. The most definitive test for polymyositis is
    A. creatine phosphokinase levels
    B. lactic dehydrogenase levels
    C. electromyography
    D. sedimentation rate
    E. muscle histology and histochemistry

12. Motor nerve conduction velocities of patients with uremic neuropathy are improved most with
    A. peritoneal dialysis
    B. hemodialysis
    C. vitamins
    D. renal transplantation
    E. A and C

13. Myasthenia gravis is
    A. associated with thymoma in 10-20% of cases
    B. more commonly associated with thymoma in males than in females
    C. more commonly associated with thymoma in young persons than in older age groups
    D. A and B
    E. B and C

14. Polymyositis usually affects which muscles initially?
    A. Lower extremity proximal muscles
    B. Lower extremity distal muscles
    C. Upper extremity proximal muscles
    D. Upper extremity distal muscles
    E. Upper and lower extremity proximal muscles

15. Paramyotonia congenita is often associated with
    A. paradoxical response to exercise
    B. bizarre high frequency potentials on EMG
    C. unusual sensitivity to cold
    D. A and B
    E. A and C

16. Neuromyotonia (Isaac's syndrome) is characterized by all the following except
    A. myokymia
    B. muscle stiffness
    C. absent sweating
    D. improvement with phenytoin
    E. equivocal improvement with quinine

17. Patients with carnitine palmityl transferase deficiency have
    A. no muscle atrophy as a rule
    B. prominent fasciculations
    C. myoglobinuria after exercise
    D. B and C
    E. A and C

18. Raynaud's phenomenon is present in approximately what percent of patients with polymyositis?
    A. 10%
    B. 30%
    C. 50%
    D. 70%
    E. 90%

19. Spontaneous pulsations of the retinal vein
    A. are present in nearly 90% of unselected patients aged 20-90
    B. are unrelated to blood pressure as a rule
    C. usually disappear at 190 mm. H_2O
    D. all of these
    E. none of these

20. Pattern-shift visual evoked responses are
    A. specific for multiple sclerosis
    B. specific for optic neuritis
    C. normal in most patients with optic neuritis
    D. all of these
    E. none of these

21. Forced downward ocular deviation is common with oculovestibular testing in patients with
    A. head injuries
    B. mass lesions
    C. sedative drug-induced coma
    D. all of these
    E. none of these

22. The blink reflex to light
    A. may be present with neocortical death despite absent visual evoked responses
    B. can be subcortically mediated
    C. has an as yet unknown afferent pathway
    D. B and C
    E. A, B and C

23. Skew deviation is most commonly due to lesions of the
    A. mesencephalon
    B. pons
    C. medulla
    D. spinal cord
    E. peripheral nerves

24. Extraocular muscle palsies associated with herpes zoster ophthalmicus are most often due to involvement of the
    A. first cranial nerve
    B. second cranial nerve
    C. third cranial nerve
    D. fourth cranial nerve
    E. sixth cranial nerve

25. Ocular myasthenia comprises what proportion of the total in Osserman's classification of myasthenia gravis?
    A. 1%
    B. 2%
    C. 5%
    D. 10%
    E. 20%

26. When temporal arteritis causes extraocular palsies, they are due to ischemia of
    A. cranial nerve III
    B. cranial nerves IV and VI
    C. the extraocular muscles
    D. the brain stem
    E. A and B

27. Pupillary light-near dissociation may be noted with
    A. Adie's pupil
    B. diabetes mellitus
    C. aberrant regeneration of the third nerve
    D. Argyll-Robertson pupils
    E. all of these

28. Clinical findings in Horner's syndrome include
    A. ptosis
    B. "upside-down" ptosis
    C. mydriasis
    D. apparent enophthalmos
    E. A, B and D

29. Opsoclonus
     A. is often continuous
     B. may be present when the eyes are closed
     C. occurs in association with neuroblastoma
     D. all of these
     E. none of these

30. A homonymous hemianopia with sparing of only the 60-
     90° portion of the temporal hemifield suggests a/an
     A. frontal lobe lesion
     B. parietal lobe lesion
     C. occipital lobe lesion
     D. optic tract lesion
     E. optic nerve lesion

31. Optic disk swelling in papilledema is chiefly due to
     A. glial swelling
     B. venous obstruction
     C. axonal swelling
     D. interstitial compartment fluid accumulation
     E. none of these

32. Clinically detectable anisocoria is present in what pro-
     portion of the population at large?
     A. 1%
     B. 5%
     C. 20%
     D. 30%
     E. 35%

33. Phenytoin and carbamazepine have both been advocated
     for treatment of focal motor and generalized epilepsy.
     A comparison of the treatments revealed
     A. no significant differences in seizure control and acute
         side effects
     B. more acute side effects with phenytoin
     C. more acute side effects with carbamazepine
     D. better seizure control with phenytoin
     E. better seizure control with carbamazepine

34. Consistent features of capsular infarcts include
     A. pure sensory loss
     B. pure motor hemiparesis
     C. hemiparesis plus homonymous hemianopsia
     D. hemiparesis with prolonged aphasia (dominant
         hemisphere)
     E. hemiparesis plus sensory loss

35. Which is the least correct statement regarding cerebral
    infarction in young adults?
    A. 25% of patients will regain functional independence
    B. hypertension and premature atherosclerosis play a
       role
    C. occlusive extracranial vascular disease in an uncom-
       mon cause
    D. cerebral embolism of cardiac origin is a frequent
       cause
    E. the etiology can be identified in over half of the cases

36. The most common location of headache in children with
    migraine is
    A. unilateral frontal
    B. bilateral frontal
    C. unilateral temporal
    D. bilateral temporal
    E. unilateral occipital

37. The most common neurologic involvement in Paget's dis-
    ease is
    A. spinal cord
    B. spinal roots and nerves
    C. cranial nerve VII
    D. cranial nerve VIII
    E. cranial nerve IX

38. Severe dementia occurs in approximately what percent
    of the population over age 65?
    A. 1%
    B. 4-5%
    C. 11-12%
    D. 17-18%
    E. 31-32%

39. In the early stages of Huntington's disease, the least
    likely feature is
    A. choreiform movements
    B. impaired short-term memory
    C. impaired retrieval from long-term memory
    D. impaired memory quotients
    E. low intelligence quotients

40. With mitral valve prolapse
    A. small strokes occur in about 5% of cases
    B. strokes, when they occur, are usually thrombotic
    C. auricular fibrillation increases the risk of embolism
    D. embolic strokes are rare
    E. none of these

41. Patients with adrenoleukodystrophy have
    A. abnormal skin pigmentation
    B. reduced adrenal reserve
    C. abnormal fatty acid synthesis
    D. A and B
    E. A, B and C

42. Hypertensive headache
    A. has a poorly understood pathogenesis
    B. represents a very small percentage of headaches in
       the general population
    C. occurs with acute hypertension
    D. occurs with chronic hypertension
    E. all of these

43. Strionigral degeneration
    A. does not respond as well to levo-dopa as does paral-
       ysis agitans
    B. may mimic Shy-Drager syndrome
    C. usually presents with a symmetrical Parkinson's
       syndrome
    D. A and B
    E. B and C

44. The neurologic complications of 5-fluorouracil therapy
    A. occur in less than 5% of patients with the usual doses
       of 15 mg/kg
    B. affect mainly the basal ganglia
    C. affect mainly the peripheral nerves
    D. are related to the total dose rather than the dose
       given at each administration
    E. C and D

45. Vincristine
    A. does not cause seizures
    B. almost always causes a peripheral neuropathy
    C. spares the autonomic nervous system as a rule
    D. has an effective antidote to minimize its toxicity
    E. all of these

46. Facial myokymia
    A. is a persistent quivering of muscles of the face
    B. is more common than myokymia of the upper extremities
    C. may be seen with polyradiculoneuropathy
    D. is often associated with multiple sclerosis or brain stem neoplasms
    E. all of these

47. Which is the least correct statement regarding anti-convulsants?
    A. Valproate is often effective for petit mal attacks
    B. Valproate is at times effective for grand mal attacks
    C. Trimethadione is usually effective for grand mal attacks
    D. Phenytoin is not predictably effective if given intra-muscularly
    E. Primidone is partially metabolized to phenobarbital

48. Which is the least correct statement regarding partial seizures with complex symptomatology?
    A. They are also known as psychomotor seizures
    B. Some of them may be temporal lobe seizures
    C. They may at times require treatment with temporal lobectomy
    D. They respond best to ethosuximide
    E. They respond about equally well to phenytoin as to carbamazepine

49. Intracranial aneurysms have the following characteristics except
    A. their prevalence has remained fairly constant
    B. they are more common in males
    C. the highest likelihood of rupture is in the sixth decade
    D. surgical treatment has been found superior to conservative management in alert patients
    E. about 2% occur in children or adolescents

50. Which statement is not true of hypertensive encephalopathy?
    A. It appears to be increasing in incidence
    B. Hypertension of whatever cause may produce it
    C. Convulsions are common with this condition
    D. Papilledema is generally related to the increase in intracranial pressure
    E. It is affecting a larger number of older patients in recent years

51. Regarding risk factors for cerebral complications of angiography for transient ischemic attacks and stroke
    A. risk is equivocally related to the number of selective injections
    B. the degree of arterial stenosis strongly affects the risk
    C. patients who need the study the most tend to be those at greatest risk from it
    D. all of these
    E. none of these

52. Primary intracerebral hemorrhage
    A. decreases after age 50
    B. is more common in males than in females
    C. has gradually decreased in incidence during the past 30 years
    D. has an incidence of about 12 per 100,000 per year in Rochester, Minnesota
    E. B, C and D

53. Phenytoin effects on bone and vitamin D metabolism may cause
    A. decrease in serum albumin
    B. increase in serum calcium
    C. decrease in serum alkaline phosphatase
    D. A and B
    E. B and C

54. A normal EEG in an unresponsive patient suggests
    A. diabetic coma
    B. ruptured basilar aneurysm
    C. hepatic encephalopathy
    D. drug overdose
    E. none of these

55. Occipital spikes on the EEG during photic stimulation
    A. are considered nonspecific
    B. correlate with visual field defects
    C. are usually seen with posterior cerebral artery infarctions
    D. are diagnostic of epilepsy
    E. none of these

56. A reversible isopotential EEG can occur in
   A. hepatic encephalopathy
   B. glioblastoma multiforme
   C. hyperthermia
   D. hypothermia
   E. C and D

57. EEG alpha rhythm in a comatose patient implies
   A. certain imminent death
   B. slight possibility of recovery
   C. probably recovery with neurologic deficit
   D. permanent vegetative state
   E. full recovery

58. Which statement is most correct concerning the EEG of patients with multiple sclerosis?
   A. It is diagnostic
   B. It is almost always normal
   C. The abnormalities are nonspecific
   D. It usually shows seizure discharges
   E. It shows focal delta near plaques

59. Unilateral μ rhythm in the EEG
   A. does not occur as an isolated finding
   B. implies ipsilateral disease
   C. implies contralateral disease
   D. is normal
   E. has no significance

60. The most common EEG abnormality in hydrocephalus is
   A. asynchronous sleep activity
   B. lateralized suppression
   C. spike-wave patterns
   D. diffuse delta
   E. diffuse theta

61. EEG seizure discharges tend to be activated by
   A. alcohol
   B. sugar
   C. milk
   D. A and B
   E. B and C

62. The EEG in rage attacks generally shows
   A. no change
   B. anterior temporal spikes
   C. mesial temporal sharp waves
   D. diffuse temporal theta
   E. diffuse temporal delta

63. 14 and 6/sec. positive spikes on the EEG correlate with
   A. lupus erythematosus
   B. middle cerebral artery aneurysms
   C. ichthyosis
   D. autonomic disturbances
   E. syphilis

64. The EEG changes in pernicious anemia correlate best with
   A. serum B_{12} levels
   B. the degree of anemia
   C. the degree of cerebral dysfunction
   D. the degree of bone marrow changes
   E. none of these

65. Accurate prediction of post-traumatic seizures following head trauma can be made if the EEG
   A. contains seizure discharges
   B. is diffusely slow
   C. contains focal slowing
   D. is normal
   E. none of these

66. Normal EEG's in patients with senile dementia are seen in
   A. 0%
   B. 20%
   C. 40%
   D. 60%
   E. 80%

67. Complete recovery from the state of electrocerebral silence, as properly defined, may occur with
   A. hepatic encephalopathy
   B. glioblastoma multiforme
   C. head trauma
   D. drug overdose
   E. epidural hematoma

68. Chronic alcohol ingestion often causes which EEG changes?
    A. Small sharp spikes
    B. Excessive photic sensitivity
    C. Excessive "build-up" on hyperventilation
    D. Diffuse slow rhythms
    E. B and D

69. Infantile spasms are associated with which EEG pattern?
    A. Multifocal spikes and slow waves
    B. Anterior temporal sharp waves
    C. Diffuse rhythmic fast spikes
    D. 3/sec. spike and wave
    E. None of these

70. A patient with uremic encephalopathy has diffuse delta slowing of his EEG. His clinical state most likely is
    A. alert
    B. confused
    C. delirious
    D. comatose
    E. clinical death

71. The EEG changes from high doses of intravenous penicillin may be
    A. focal spikes
    B. focal delta slowing
    C. diffuse slowing
    D. diffuse spike-wave discharges
    E. sleep apnea

72. During an attack of periodic paralysis, the EMG typically shows
    A. marked polyphasic activity
    B. single unit interference pattern with short duration action potentials
    C. fibrillation potentials
    D. "dive-bomber" discharges
    E. electrical silence

73. Extremely periodic EEG bursts of sharp and slow activity in a child with dementia suggest
    A. Krabbe's disease
    B. SSPE
    C. metachromatic leukodystrophy
    D. juvenile Huntington's disease
    E. Hallervorden-Spatz disease

74. The storage material which accumulates in metachromatic leukodystrophy
    A. results from a deficiency of arylsulfatase A
    B. is a breakdown product of abnormal myelin
    C. is found principally in oligodendrocytes of cerebral white matter
    D. all of these
    E. none of these

75. The most important single factor in producing radiation myelopathy is
    A. high total dose
    B. high fraction size
    C. shorter treatment time
    D. longer treatment time
    E. increased length of cord treated

76. Which is not a feature of the cerebrohepatorenal syndrome of Zellweger?
    A. Failure to thrive
    B. Early death
    C. Marked hypertonia
    D. Abnormal facies
    E. Psychomotor retardation

77. Which structure is pathologically involved in Wernicke's encephalopathy but not in subacute necrotizing encephalomyelitis?
    A. Cerebellum
    B. Basal ganglia
    C. Spinal cord
    D. Mammillary bodies
    E. Walls of the third ventricle

78. Spinal arachnoiditis
    A. is a focal process pathologically as a rule
    B. is most common below the age of 20
    C. is as common as intraspinal tumors
    D. usually presents with nerve root pain
    E. none of these

79. Peroxisomes are deficient in
    A. Fabry's disease
    B. Pelizaeus-Merzbacher disease
    C. the cerebrohepatorenal syndrome
    D. the ataxia-telangiectasia syndrome
    E. peroxide poisoning

80. N-hexane toxicity
    A. may occur from addictive glue-sniffing
    B. is primarily a motor neuropathy
    C. is a giant axonal neuropathy
    D. A and C
    E. A and B

81. The most common intraspinal tumors are
    A. meningiomas and neurofibromas
    B. meningiomas and ependymomas
    C. ependymomas and sarcomas
    D. neurofibromas and sarcomas
    E. meningiomas and sarcomas

82. Almost pure axonal degeneration in peripheral nerves is produced by
    A. lead
    B. triethyl tin
    C. diphtheria toxin
    D. acrylamide
    E. all of these

83. Whipple's disease
    A. is caused by a virus
    B. is a reversible metabolic disorder
    C. is a lipid storage disorder which usually involves the CNS
    D. is caused by a parasite
    E. may present with only CNS symptoms

84. The least correct statement concerning medulloepitheliomas is they
    A. are highly malignant
    B. are common neoplasms
    C. occur in early childhood
    D. are common in the cerebrum
    E. involve the CNS

85. Which substance does not usually cause human toxic distal axonopathy?
    A. N-hexane
    B. Disulfiram
    C. Mercury
    D. Isoniazid
    E. Nitrofurantoin

86. The pathophysiology of myasthenia gravis is now thought to be
    A. hypersensitivity to acetylcholine
    B. hyposensitivity to acetylcholine
    C. decreased number of acetylcholine receptors
    D. reduced number of acetylcholine quanta
    E. reduced number of acetylcholine molecules per quanta

87. The peak effect of amantadine in parkinsonism occurs
    A. in the first week
    B. at 6 months
    C. at one year
    D. at two years
    E. at three years

88. Which of the following drug categories can be related to increased EEG beta rhythm?
    A. Ethanol
    B. Benzodiazepines
    C. Antihistamines
    D. Tricyclics
    E. All of these

89. Which of the following are dopamine agonists?
    A. Amphetamine
    B. Levo-dopa
    C. Bromocriptine
    D. All of these
    E. B and C only

90. Postanoxic intention myoclonus may respond to
    A. benzodiazepines
    B. 5-hydroxytryptophan
    C. valproic acid
    D. all of these
    E. none of these

91. Anticonvulsants restore presynaptic inhibition by releasing
    A. cyclic nucleotides
    B. high energy phosphate compounds
    C. inhibitory neurotransmitters
    D. excitatory neurotransmitters
    E. none of these

92.   Organophosphate poisoning may be reversed by
        A. nicotine
        B. physostigmine
        C. atropine
        D. PAM (pyridine-2-aldoxime)
        E. all of these

93.   The blood transketolase assay helps to detect
        A. ATP deficiency
        B. niacin deficiency
        C. thiamine deficiency
        D. cyclic AMP deficiency
        E. none of these

94.   The majority of the optic tract receives its blood supply
        from the
        A. posterior communicating artery
        B. posterior cerebral artery
        C. posterior choroidal artery
        D. anterior choroidal artery
        E. none of these

95.   Sodium valproate
        A. lowers whole-brain GABA levels
        B. depolarizes the resting membrane potential
        C. is a poor anticonvulsant
        D. all of these
        E. none of these

96.   All the following favor meningioma over acoustic neu-
        roma, with a cerebellopontine mass demonstrated on CT
        scan except
        A. round shape
        B. increased attenuation
        C. marked calcification
        D. widening of porus
        E. center of tumor anterior to the internal acoustic
            meatus

97.   The most helpful computerized tomography finding to dis-
        tinguish Dandy-Walker syndrome from arachnoid cyst is
        A. obstructive hydrocephalus
        B. elevation of the transverse sinus
        C. hypoplasia of the cerebellar vermis and hemispheres
        D. demonstration of a CSF density midline cyst which
            does not displace the cerebellum
        E. none of these

98. Which is the <u>least</u> common mass lesion seen in the sup-
    rasellar cistern on CT scan?
    A. Hypothalamic glioma
    B. Meningioma
    C. Aneurysm
    D. Pituitary adenoma
    E. Craniopharyngioma

99. <u>Remote</u> head trauma may produce all the following CT
    patterns <u>except</u>
    A. porencephaly
    B. cerebral edema
    C. subdural hematoma
    D. communicating hydrocephalus
    E. post-traumatic infarct (closed porencephaly)

100. Microcephaly is <u>not</u> produced by
    A. neonatal cere<u>br</u>al ischemia
    B. intra-uterine infection
    C. mucopolysaccharidoses
    D. post-meningoencephalitis
    E. hereditary micrencephaly of Penrose

POST-TEST ANSWER KEY

1.	A	37.	D	73.	B
2.	C	38.	B	74.	A
3.	E	39.	E	75.	B
4.	B	40.	C	76.	C
5.	D	41.	D	77.	D
6.	D	42.	E	78.	D
7.	B	43.	D	79.	C
8.	E	44.	A	80.	D
9.	B	45.	B	81.	A
10.	C	46.	E	82.	D
11.	E	47.	C	83.	E
12.	D	48.	D	84.	B
13.	D	49.	B	85.	C
14.	A	50.	A	86.	C
15.	E	51.	D	87.	A
16.	C	52.	E	88.	B
17.	E	53.	A	89.	D
18.	B	54.	E	90.	D
19.	D	55.	A	91.	C
20.	E	56.	E	92.	D
21.	C	57.	B	93.	C
22.	E	58.	C	94.	D
23.	B	59.	B	95.	E
24.	C	60.	A	96.	A
25.	E	61.	A	97.	C
26.	C	62.	A	98.	A
27.	E	63.	D	99.	B
28.	E	64.	C	100.	C
29.	D	65.	E		
30.	C	66.	B		
31.	C	67.	D		
32.	C	68.	E		
33.	A	69.	A		
34.	B	70.	D		
35.	A	71.	C		
36.	B	72.	E		